Nellie A. Radomsky, MD, I...

Lost Voices:
Women, Chronic Pain, and Abuse

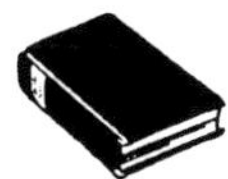

Pre-publication
REVIEWS,
COMMENTARIES,
EVALUATIONS . . .

"A sensitive and compassionate young physician writes from the vantage of her own struggle, a struggle to move beyond 'diagnosis and cure' to hearing the lost voices of women in pain. Through the stories of Sharon and Anna and others the reader is gently but purposefully guided through the complexity of chronic pain to begin the healing process. Dr. Radomsky speaks of 'Hermedicine,' a form of medicine in which the female experience is validated and empowerment is nourished. As a woman, a health professional or a counselor you will find insights and encouragement in this book."

Marlene Reimer, RN
Associate Professor of Nursing,
The University of Calgary

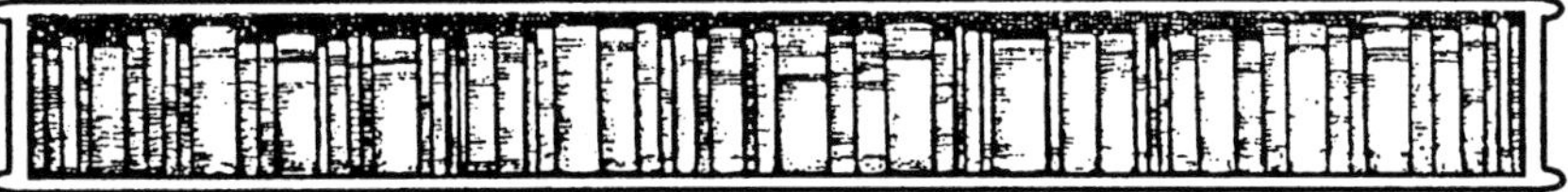

More pre-publication
REVIEWS, COMMENTARIES, EVALUATIONS . . .

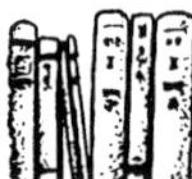

"I found this a very moving, engaging, and important book. In fact I read it in two sittings. In spite of my reluctance to read again about these painful problems, I couldn't put it down.

Dr. Radomsky uses simple, direct language about a complex, costly problem that robs some women of themselves and their many potential contributions to society. This book brings for all of us new understandings about health care and the doctor/patient relationship.

Dr. Radomsky allows her patients to tell us their stories, and in so doing, she demonstrates for us a new kind of humane and caring physician.

This book is for all women–women who have hurt, women who care for women, and all health professionals, male and female."

Susan H. McDaniel, PhD
Associate Professor of Psychiatry
and Family Medicine,
University of Rochester
and Highland Hospital

"*Lost Voices* brings feminist theory to life through down-to-earth stories that will bring new insights to every woman whether or not she suffers from chronic illness. Dr. Radomsky dramatically reveals the debilitating effects of the repression of women, but at the same time inspirits us with the stories of her patients' courageous efforts to reclaim their own truth. This is a book with heart.

By helping her patients reclaim their own voices, Dr. Radomsky discovers her own voice as a woman physician. Her creative and uniquely feminine approach to the puzzle of chronic pain is like a breath of fresh air, a welcome relief from the often lifeless and sterile world of medical science.

Dr. Radomsky demystifies the doctor/patient relationship and lays the groundwork for caring partnership. I highly recommend this book not only for consumers of health care, but for every health care professional who wants to learn how to care as well as to cure."

Carol Montgomery, RN, PhD
Author of *Healing Through Communication: The Practice of Caring*

More pre-publication
REVIEWS, COMMENTARIES, EVALUATIONS . . .

"Nellie Radomsky's *Lost Voices* cries out from a medical wilderness that for too long has failed to comprehend the unique interplay between the psychology of women and the inadequacies of a medical system that is purely mechanistic. With heart and unqualified technical competence, Dr. Radomsky has crafted a book that should not only be required reading for all physicians, but that will also touch the soul of any woman who has survived physical or sexual abuse or who has endured chronic pain within a medical system that knows little about women, pain, or abuse.

Lost Voices is as balanced as any work of its kind could ever be, and then some. The chapters on medical research and incidence of abuse and chronic pain are solid without putting the reader to sleep. The case studies are poignant and powerful, sad and uplifting. Throughout her work, Dr. Radomsky displays the compassion, sensitivity, and obvious depth of knowledge that anyone, man or woman, would hope to find in a physician. My only hope is that this book finds its way into the hands of thousands of doctors and patients who have struggled together to understand the causes of each others' discomfort."

Linda D. Friel, MA
Licensed Psychologist;
Author of *Adult Children: The Secrets of Dysfunctional Families*

Harrington Park Press
An Imprint of The Haworth Press, Inc.

NOTES FOR PROFESSIONAL LIBRARIANS AND LIBRARY USERS

This is an original book title published by Harrington Park Press, an imprint of The Haworth Press, Inc. Unless otherwise noted in specific chapters with attribution, materials in this book have not been previously published elsewhere in any format or language.

CONSERVATION AND PRESERVATION NOTES

All books published by The Haworth Press, Inc. and its imprints are printed on certified ph neutral, acid free book grade paper. This paper meets the minimum requirements of American National Standard for Information Sciences–Permanence of Paper for Printed Material, ANSI Z39.48-1984.

Lost Voices
Women, Chronic Pain, and Abuse

THE HAWORTH PRESS
New, Recent, and Forthcoming Titles
of Related Interest

Prisoners of Ritual: An Odyssey into Female Genital Circumcision in Africa by Hanny Lightfoot-Klein

Waiting: A Diary of Loss and Hope in Pregnancy by Ellen Judith Reich

Women and Aging: Celebrating Ourselves by Ruth Raymond Thone

Women's Conflicts about Eating and Sexuality by Rosalyn Meadow/Lillie Weiss

A Woman's Odyssey into Africa: Tracks Across a Life by Hanny Lightfoot-Klein

Tending Inner Gardens: The Healing Art of Feminist Psychotherapy by Lesley Irene Shore

The Way of the Woman Writer by Janet Lynn Roseman

Lost Voices
Women, Chronic Pain, and Abuse

Nellie A. Radomsky, MD, PhD

Harrington Park Press
An Imprint of The Haworth Press, Inc.
New York • London

Published by

Harrington Park Press, an imprint of The Haworth Press, Inc., 10 Alice Street, Binghamton, NY 13904-1580

Library of Congress Cataloging-in-Publication Data

Radomsky, Nellie A.
Lost voices : women, chronic pain, and abuse / Nellie A. Radomsky.
p. cm.
Includes bibliographical references and index.
ISBN 1-56023-864-X (acid-free paper : pbk.)
1. Chronic pain. 2. Women–Health and hygiene. 3. Abused women–Health and hygiene. 4. Abused women–Mental health. 5. Chronic pain–Psychological aspects. I. Title.
RB127.R33 1995
616'.0472'082–dc20 94-29611
CIP

To Alena Marie

ABOUT THE AUTHOR

Nellie Radomsky, MD, PhD, a family physician with 16 years experience, is in private practice in Red Deer, Alberta, Canada. She also serves as Clinical Assistant Professor of Family Medicine at the University of Calgary. In addition to her clinical work, she conducts workshops and has presented papers on abuse and chronic pain at national and international medical conferences. Currently, Dr. Radomsky is involved in research on physician education about abuse issues. She is a member of the College of Family Physicians of Canada and the Society of Teachers of Family Medicine, and a member of the Board of Trustees of the Alberta Heritage Foundation for Medical Research.

CONTENTS

Preface

I wrote this book for all women who experience chronic pain and for all women who feel silenced. I wrote for women who sit patiently in doctor's offices hoping to be fixed. I wrote for women who feel confused when more blood tests, more X rays, more procedures, and more knives put into their bodies fail to remove pain.

This book began, although I did not realize it at the time, with a small research project conducted in my office. The research project grew out of the confusion I experienced when women with chronic pain refused to get better–when they refused to comply with my presumed superior knowledge. The project represented my struggle to understand why it was that women staying in the women's shelter inevitably had stories of chronic pain and many surgeries along with the stories of abuse–why it was that women with chronic pain often had complex and abusive past histories.

My training emphasized "diagnosis and cure." My training taught me to objectify patients and encouraged reductionistic and cause-and-effect thinking. This approach did not prepare me for the world of women and chronic pain.

These pages reflect my struggle. I gradually learned to listen to women who trusted me enough to share their stories. I began to see the ways I too had been silenced on personal and professional levels. To these women, who came to my office and challenged me and continued to see me, I am grateful. They continue to teach me to move beyond diagnostic labels.

In this book, I describe the complexity of chronic pain as experienced by women and provide evidence for an association with abuse issues. In the first part, I explore chronic pain from the perspective of current medical practice and how issues of abuse remain largely unrecognized by medical practitioners, or, more precisely, how women are silenced in the doctor's office. Historical and cultural issues as they pertain to medical models and the doctor-patient relationship are also addressed.

In the second part, I explore the sense of the lost voices of women in pain. I do this by creating stories based on themes repeatedly told to me in the office. This leads to the final section where I continue in a narrative fashion to explore the healing process. *Lost Voices* is a guide for women to unseen and unknown restraints dictated by personal history and the culture. It is a guide for understanding the complexity of chronic pain and how finding the lost voice can begin the healing process.

It is my hope that the book will encourage women who are in pain to give voice to their buried experiences. I hope that both care givers and those they care for will be inspired to search for new meaning in chronic pain stories and will be challenged to move beyond simplistic diagnostic labels.

Acknowledgements

There are those whose encouragement and willingness to be in conversation with me proved vital to the completion of this book. There are many contributors and to all of you I am deeply grateful. To the women who shared their stories with me in my office–I thank you. It continues to be a privilege for me to be trusted by people who share their pain and joy. Many of you are my best teachers.

I would also like to thank: Gwen Hopkins, who consistently laughed and cried with me; Betty Cowie, who listened, conversed, and cared; Esmie Tyson, Madeline Sparrow, Susan Wong, Virginia Nemetz, and Marcella Barthel, who read parts of the book and enthusiastically helped me clarify my work; Joanne Jarvis and Barb Slater, who understood those days when my clinical work slowed down; Sigmund Brouwer, who helped me begin to write, even when I emphatically insisted that it was impossible; my sisters–Carol Nicks, Shirley Freed, Patsy Trefz, and Ingrid Ostrem–who love me and endlessly share ideas with me; Alena Radomsky, who gives me joy and happiness; and John Radomsky, for his support.

Introduction

> In traditional American biomedicine, the typical physician-patient relationship has been characterized by the patient offering a description of symptoms and their history, together with his or her body for examination and laboratory tests, to the physician who adduces the definitive "clinical picture"–the official story–from it. From this story, the physician recommends a course of action, with which the patient is expected to comply, thereby completing the physician's story as it "should" unfold. The patient's (and patient's family's and community's) own story is, in this official biomedical framework, incidental even if interesting. For the most part, patients' stories are viewed as signs of ignorance, bizarre or quaint thinking, or sheer mental illness–in any event, to be circumvented and not to be taken seriously except as obstacles to the completeness of the physician's own story.
>
> –Stein and Apprey, *Clinical Stories and Their Translations*

My training in medicine 16 years ago exposed me to "diagnosis and cure" thinking in the fashion Stein and Apprey (1990) describe. I certainly experienced compartmentalized thinking. I thought about my patients in terms of "is the complaint real?"; that is, does the problem reside in the body or is the problem in the mind and somehow not so worthy of my attention? I had minimal sense of the patient and the experience of illness, but rather felt obsessed with the notion of disease. My approach was to find the disease lurking in the body and stamp out the disease. It's difficult to know for sure, but somewhere after ten years of medical practice I began to see the limitations of my approach and felt there must be a better way. Viewed from the outside, my situation looks traditional and satisfying. I practice in a clinic with 14 partners. I have privileges at a 400-bed community hospital. My practice includes obstetrics. I have attracted considerably more women to my practice than men and it really is the women in my practice who began to challenge my approach.

These women challenged me in many ways, but mostly because their chronic pain problems persisted and they refused to get better. At first I blamed them. They just lacked initiative. They could get better if they just tried. Eventually my own pain forced me to take another look at old assumptions and old ideas. The door gradually opened to new ways of thinking about many of these women and myself.

In medicine, there is a bias toward understanding disease at the biological and biochemical level only. This reductionistic tendency, however, seemed to be just part of the problem. Of equal concern was my own biased approach to women and many of their health issues.

Had I studied medicine or "Hismedicine?" My own view of women as more passive, more demanding, more neurotic, more prone to bodily aches and pains of a minor nature, and thus inferior and somehow lacking, was not an idea I readily acknowledged. Yet I think it existed. After all, how could I have escaped stereotypical ideas prevalent in medicine? Certainly most would agree that the current practice of medicine thrives on hierarchical power structures. Had my training in medicine encouraged me to think for myself or to question traditional ideas? Mostly I learned to "help" and to conform, which for my women patients too often translated as, "trust my expert opinion–distrust your own body and your own ideas."

At some point, it occurred to me that what I needed was a greater sense of "Hermedicine." Instead of always judging the female against an assumed normal male, it seemed time to recognize the female experience and her expertise about her own body. Should not her illness and disease be understood within the context of the culture?

During this transition period many people influenced me. However, it was mainly women patients who shared stories and gave me new insights. (The word patient has limitations but I will use it throughout this book.) In the midst of this change I focused more on women with chronic pain. My effort to put these women into tightly defined categories regularly failed. In addition, I realized I was not connecting with them in a meaningful way. Eventually I stopped trying to make the correct diagnosis when it came to these chronic pain problems that had no identifiable organic cause. I started listening and asked different questions. As I altered my obsession with cure for chronic pain, I began to notice some changes. Many of these women started to talk to me about their lives. Some told painful and disturbing stories. I didn't want to hear about abuse and neglect. Gradually these women taught me how to listen. This new path eventually took me into my own research project on chronic pain and abuse (Radomsky, 1992). I will briefly summarize the results.

In my study of 120 women from my practice, I found that women who identified alcohol-dependent or harsh, rigid, or difficult parents were at increased risk for chronic illnesses, most of which were chronic pain problems. In addition these women reported more sexual and/or physical abuse (32% and 44%, respectively) than women who denied having parents with these characteristics (8%). Women identifying abuse (23% overall) were diagnosed with more chronic illness (67%, compared with 25%) and more lifetime surgeries (3.3, compared with 1.75) than women denying abuse. The women in the study were relatively young (mean age of 34) and 81% of the women had a 12th grade education or greater. All women were white except for one Native American and one Asian. Men were excluded from the study only because my practice is predominantly female, and with limited funding I was in no position to embark on a study outside my practice.

The degree to which chronic illness and frequency of surgeries were associated with abuse surprised me. My training had focused on the relationship between abuse and psychiatric illness, or abuse and overt physical injury. Certainly the association between abuse and chronic illness is recognized, but as a physician I don't think I behaved as if I believed the connection.

While conducting my research and subsequent to completing the project, I gradually realized the connection between chronic pain and powerlessness in women. Women who told stories about abuse always told stories in which they were silenced. Women identifying rigid and difficult or alcohol-dependent parents inevitably experienced loss of their own voice in these family systems. Their families reinforced helplessness–sometimes by overt abuse, but also through continual invalidation. It was particularly painful for me to realize the degree to which I had labeled women neurotic, inadequate, or helpless with no sense of the degree to which they were frightened, frustrated, angry, dehumanized, and regularly the victims of violence. My research revealed extensive victimization of women in the family. In addition, I realized the ways these women were often victimized again in the community.

Many women said to me: "Why can't you write something for us?" I realized that my research paper addressed only part of what I had experienced. Eventually I understood my reasons for this book.

I recognize that powerlessness and chronic pain can be issues for men as well. However, I've chosen to limit the discussion to women. Issues for men and women may overlap, since men too are victims of abuse and violence, but the very nature of the Western patriarchal culture dictates power to men. The role women play far too often becomes determined by men. The patriarchal system encourages the development of self-sufficiency, power, and the rational mind for men and delegates to women the role of developing more intuitive skills–perception, emotional responsiveness, and nurturing. Paradoxically, powerlessness for men in this culture often translates into violent behavior, alcoholism, and antisocial behavior. Developing a more integrated self, with a sense of inner power that allows a greater sense of mutual empowerment, will therefore have different meaning for women and minorities than for many men.

I begin the book with a story about chronic pain, abuse, and healing. The story on its own seems straightforward. However, in the six chapters that follow I refer to the story and discuss some of its complexities. This allows me to explore with the reader how doctors and patients think and talk about pain.

I begin Chapter 2 with a discussion about the magnitude of pain problems. In Chapter 3, I discuss medical models to give insight into how doctors think about pain and in turn how patients have responded. Likewise, this gives some insight into the impasse that doctors and patients experience so often when chronic pain is the issue. In Chapter 4, I continue the discussion of chronic pain and point out the differences between acute and chronic pain. I elaborate on how confusion with the diagnosis of pain problems often stems from our difficulty in understanding acute versus chronic pain issues. This leads to the discussion in Chapter 5 of chronic pain experienced by women. I focus on chronic pain problems where there is no readily identified organic explanation for the pain. I suggest that the traditional medical approach does not allow for the meaning of the chronic pain symptoms women experience to emerge in the clinical setting. This leads to a discussion in Chapter 6 on culture and gender in medicine. I conclude the first section with a summary of the medical literature that suggests an association between chronic pain problems that women experience and abuse. I review the few research papers that address the present approach of physicians with respect to domestic violence issues. I raise concerns about the present medical research agenda that may not perceive issues with psychosocial and behavioral concerns–such as sexual assault, domestic violence, eating disorders, and chronic pain problems with no identifiable organic cause–as legitimate and important areas of medical research. I suggest that while women wait for the medical community to hear their concerns, they might begin to hear each other. This discussion leads to the stories in Part II. Readers may find some of the information in Part I tedious, although I have tried to minimize the use of medical jargon. Readers may choose to begin with the stories in Part II and refer to Part I for specific information.

In Part II, I make a shift in terms of how the information is presented. In the first part I really ask readers to think with me. In Part II, I ask readers to move into greater awareness of their emotional responses. I do this by simply sharing stories of women in chronic pain who also identify abuse of some sort.

I begin with a historical story–the sense of a lost voice in the "herstory" of "Hismedicine." I follow with six contemporary stories. All of the women in these stories are fictional. I created them to carry the accounts of personal stories of pain that many women shared with me. By reconstructing in this form I have protected women in my practice. I've made no attempt to be inclusive in terms of chronic pain problems. The chronic pain problems I focus on are those in which the pain is not related to readily identifiable organic disease, but rather is thought to have psychophysiologic origins. Women seem particularly prone to that type of pain problem. I've chosen common situations as observed in my practice that typify women and their chronic pain. In each case, I tell the story and reflect on it as I do. I think out loud while relating the story, and these thoughts are included in italics. In so doing I hope to encourage readers to become aware of their own feelings and ideas. In this way I hope to explore with the reader and together find greater understanding of women and chronic pain.

The book concludes in Part III with a discussion about chronic pain and the healing journey. In this section, I again refer to the original story of chronic pain and abuse. I focus in Chapter 15 on some concerns women may have as they address their chronic pain problems. I suggest practical approaches and include information about seeking professional care. In Chapter 16, I reflect on issues that are not so obvious with chronic pain and healing. I include experiences with women that have helped me begin to understand that healing from chronic pain is about empowering women to become who they are. The final chapter is another story–a story about the lost voice of the feminine and a glimpse of one healing journey.

I recognize that I seem to be suggesting that I speak for all women. I understand that this is not the case. I emphasize that my contribution reflects my background, my color, and my sexual preference.

My father's parents came to Canada from Sweden in 1912. My mother's parents were from a western European background and came to Canada from Nebraska in the early 1900s. I grew up with my parents, siblings, and many relatives on a farm in central Alberta.

My stories and ideas reflect this background. Also, because of my concern to be as accurate as possible, I have included stories in which the themes were repeatedly told to me. Ultimately, the stories are my interpretation. I've portrayed myself as honestly as possible to reinforce my own conviction that the doctor-patient relationship is, after all, an engagement between two humans, in which both struggle for the miracle and meaning of life itself.

REFERENCES

Radomsky, N.A. (1992). The association of parental alcoholism and rigidity with chronic illness and abuse among women. *J Fam Pract* 35:54-60.

Stein, H.F. and Apprey, M. (1990). *Clinical Stories and Their Translations.* Vol. 3 in the Series in Ethnicity, Medicine and Psychoanalysis (p. 8). Charlottesville: University of Virginia.

PART I. CHRONIC PAIN: THE REALITY OF WHAT HURTS

I have a pain in my womb. It doesn't go away. Two doctors say I must have a hysterectomy. My response is stoical, but I have bad dreams.

–Sylvia Fraser, *My Father's House*

Chapter 1

Flying Bricks

> I'm sorry there is so much pain in this story. I'm sorry it's in fragments, like a body caught in crossfire or pulled apart by force. But there is nothing I can do to change it.
>
> –Margaret Atwood, *The Handmaid's Tale*

SHARON'S STORY

The First Visit

I glanced at my watch as I hurriedly walked past the waiting room to my office. An hour behind. I groaned inwardly. I knew this frustrated everyone. I could hear the noise from the waiting room. Babies crying. Adults coughing. Mothers talking to their children. But today had been one of those days. Babies enter the world when they are ready. I could still feel my own excitement about the delivery. Everything went okay–that was always a big relief. But the timing meant confusion and I knew I'd spend the remainder of the afternoon struggling to catch up.

I quickly got organized and started seeing patients. The afternoon progressed. And then I noticed that the chart for the next patient was thin. A new patient–hopefully this wouldn't be complicated. Sharon Thompson–born 1949. I opened the door and quickly introduced myself. My examining rooms are arranged with a small desk-type counter that allows me to sit next to the patient rather than across from them. This means I don't feel as if I'm talking across a barrier.

Sharon looked at me intently and then launched into a story about pain in her body. As she talked I sensed she tossed bricks about the room. The bricks weren't aimed at me personally. But the bricks were labeled. Inadequate doctors. Insensitive doctors. Bad doctors. I hate doctors. Why can't doctors help me? Doctors frustrate me. If I could I would get rid of all doctors. The bricks flew in all directions. I knew there was no point in trying to stop the bricks. I sat there and wished for a bigger room. I imagined moving my chair behind the desk. I nodded occasionally and watched bricks hit my walls. After eight minutes of this she gradually slowed the pace and then said, "But I'm seeing you because my friend Jane comes here and she thought you could help me with this pain."

By now her physical presence had fully registered. Sharon was not a big woman. She was small, otherwise I may have already escaped. Thin, straight brown hair framed a face with no makeup and intense sharp eyes. Her clothes were regular–the things you wear about the house–blue jeans and an old white sweat shirt.

"Yes, I see you have pain and are upset, Sharon," I responded quickly, relieved that the bricks had stopped flying.

She relaxed ever so little and looked at me expectantly.

"But your problem sounds big to me and I doubt that we'll find an easy answer. In fact, Sharon, I think we'd first best figure out how we might work together."

She looked confused and disappointed.

"What do you mean? Jane said you could help me."

"The way I see things, Sharon, you've had pain for at least twenty years. You've seen many doctors. You've had many tests and furthermore you've had a lot of operations. I gather you've avoided doctors with hospital privileges for that reason."

She nodded.

"So it seems to me that we might try something different."

She waited.

"I'm sure I don't know any magic tests and I suspect you've had every type of drug in the book."

"But my neck and back hurt so much–do you mean you can't help me?"

"No, I just think we first need to figure out how we'll work together. What I mean is that you and I will both need to work on understanding this pain stuff and will both need to try a different approach."

She continued to look bewildered.

"I suggest, Sharon, that you think about what I'm saying. If you want to see me again I'd like you to book for a complete checkup. I think I need to see you when I have more time to address your problems. I need to get to know you and I want both of us to be trying to understand this pain problem. I just don't think after all these years of you trying to get doctors to solve this pain and clearly not getting anywhere that we'll likely find a simple easy answer."

"So what do I do in the meantime?"

"Well, first of all I'd like you to really think about what I've said. If you are willing to work together with me then I'd like you to book another appointment. And I don't know what you can do about the pain. Anything that has helped you in the past–for sure continue."

I found myself shutting her chart. I shifted and realized I had to get moving.

Sharon said, "Okay, I'll think about this."

"And don't forget to book for a complete checkup," I said.

I quickly moved to the next room hoping that the remainder of the day would be easier. I didn't think too much about Sharon. I had no idea if she'd see me again. I wasn't sure if she wanted any responsibility in addressing the pain. I knew if she returned this pain thing would be a challenge.

Four Weeks Later

Sharon returned. She had booked for a complete checkup. This time I wasn't behind. I usually feel more energetic in the morning and opened the door to the examining room with curiosity. I wondered if there would be more flying bricks.

Sharon looked less hostile, although not exactly relaxed.

"So, how have you been?"

"About the same," she said.

I noticed that she wore the same blue jeans and her thin body occupied the chair in the same pushy manner.

"What I want to do, Sharon, is get a good story, so I'll ask lots of questions and then I'll do the physical exam."

She nodded.

"So tell me about the pain?"

"I hurt mostly in my neck and upper back. Sometimes I get headaches. I think I hurt most of the time but some days are worse than others. The pain never leaves."

"Do you think anything makes the pain worse or better?"

"Oh, I don't know. I had that physiotherapy a few years ago. I think it helped a bit, but as soon as I stopped I was quickly back to the same pain stuff."

I reviewed her previous investigations and she signed a release so I could get old records. I didn't want to repeat unnecessary investigations.

Her past history was a story of surgeries: appendectomy, tubal ligation, dilatation and curettage (she thought perhaps eight), and finally a hysterectomy.

"I ask many questions about the family," I said as I continued taking her history.

She spent her childhood on a farm in central Alberta. Both parents were alive, although the marriage had dissolved when Sharon was 15. There were five children–two boys and three girls. Sharon was the youngest. She thought all of them were basically healthy, although it didn't sound as if she saw her siblings or parents very often. There was no family history of breast cancer, heart disease, or diabetes. Her grandfather had arthritis. Sharon had married and had three daughters. Her marriage ended in divorce after four years and she raised her children alone. Presently Sharon lived alone and worked in the housekeeping department of a hotel.

"Sharon," I continued, "I routinely ask everyone about alcoholism. Were you ever concerned about your parents' use of drugs or alcohol?"

"Funny you should ask," she said. "My mother drank. So did my father, although not as much. That's why they're divorced. Actually my father doesn't drink anymore. He got married again but my mother's in deep trouble. That's why I don't visit her. I can't stand it."

"Ummmm," I murmured, "that doesn't sound good."

"No. It was a mess," she continued. "And my husband drank too. That's why I'm divorced. But I never touch the stuff."

"Uh, uh," I paused, and then continued asking questions while thinking that I would explore this more. "I ask everyone this question, Sharon. Did you experience any physical or sexual abuse while growing up or abuse in your marriage?"

She seemed to look more intently at me. Unlike many of my patients she showed no sign of anxiety.

"Oh, yes. There was sexual abuse growing up–mother's boyfriends were after me all the time and physical abuse from parents, ex-husband–and a few bad affairs. But that's all in the past."

I sensed my own anxiety. Sharon looked at me as if to say, "So–get on with it. What's this got to do with anything? I came to talk about my pain, not this stuff."

"Have you ever discussed this with anyone?" I asked.

"Oh, yes. I've gone the therapy route. All that shit has been sorted out. I was in that group program for two years–you know that group program." I nodded realizing that she had been in a group I was familiar with and had confidence in. She continued. "I wasn't the worst case but my story was right up there. But it helped me. I'm glad I finally got help for that stuff."

"Sounds like you've worked through a lot of issues, Sharon."

"Oh, yes. You can say that."

"Have you talked to any doctors about this?"

"Of course not," she said. "Doctors aren't interested in this stuff. You people don't want to know about messy stuff."

I felt stunned. "Of course we are," I thought, but realized Sharon had just shared her reality.

"Well, Sharon," I said carefully, "I suppose we doctors don't often indicate that we think these issues are relevant. But I guess I ask this because I've come to understand that these abuse issues can affect us in many ways we don't really understand."

This time Sharon looked surprised.

"What do you mean?"

"Well, it seems to me that many of my patients who have stories about abuse also have stories of unexplained medical problems. I really don't understand all of this either, but sometimes I think we just don't know what happens to us when we experience sexual, physical, emotional, or any kind of abuse."

She seemed to be thinking. "Could be."

"Anyway, Sharon," I continued, "you've worked through many issues–if you need to talk more, let me know. I'm not sure what difference it makes that you told me about the abuse. I guess I just know you better and I support you for your tremendous personal growth."

This time she said, "Ummmm."

We finished the history and then I did a physical examination. I reviewed her past tests and talked about her problem.

"From what I can figure out so far, Sharon, I think you have a type of arthritis."

"What do you mean?"

"Well, I'm not completely sure yet, but from your story, check up, and the tests you've had you look like you have fibromyalgia. That's just a fancy name for a type of pain problem that tends to affect your back, neck, and other parts of your body. People have these tender points just like you do. The frustrating thing is that the problem isn't understood very well. There are no clear tests to diagnose the problem and no easy solutions."

"So–what am I supposed to do?"

"Well, I think we need to talk about things you can do to take very good care of yourself. And sometimes physiotherapy and medication can help."

I talked about simple exercises like walking and questioned her about life-style issues. She thought she could try a few changes but she didn't want pills and didn't want to go to physiotherapy. I wanted to repeat a couple of blood tests and told her to come back in three weeks so we could review things. I hoped by then to have any significant past records.

Three Weeks Later

I no longer expected flying bricks. On this visit she looked relaxed.

"I feel better," she said.

"So what's different?"

"Well, I'm walking more. And I've been thinking–I think you're right about the pain and abuse stuff."

"What do you mean?" I realized I felt confused.

"Well, I always thought the abuse had something to do with my pain," she continued, looking excited, "but every time I saw a doctor they just kept looking for something so I kept thinking that there must be something terribly wrong with my body. But I think maybe the abuse is part of all of this pain stuff. You know, there has been so much pain. I always wondered about things, but doctors never asked so I thought it couldn't be connected. And I have always been so afraid–afraid that there's something terribly wrong with my body–afraid that everyone could see what's wrong with me." She looked at me, her face showing intensity and discomfort.

"Sharon, this sounds painful," I responded quickly, "but I think there is a connection and I've heard so many women say this–this thing about being afraid that there is something terribly wrong with their body as a result of the abuse."

And then we both sat there seeming to need to understand what we had both said.

Part of me felt shocked. My mind raced with images of angry doctors, all trying to avoid flying bricks, and all failing to diagnose and fix the pain.

We continued to talk and gradually I sensed that we both relaxed. Sharon kept seeming more powerful as she talked about changes she wanted to make, changes that had to do with Sharon taking care of Sharon.

And then we talked about her results and past tests and again concluded that she had fibromyalgia. I suggested that she return in a month so we could reassess the pain situation. She agreed.

Four Months Later

Sharon returned four months later to get her sore ears and throat checked–she had a particularly bad cold. I checked her and concluded that she really needed an antibiotic because her ear drums were red. But I also realized Sharon seemed different. This time I needed to spend more time with her.

"Sharon, can we just talk a little more? I feel I need to understand some things better."

"Sure."

"It's just that you look so much better today, Sharon, in spite of your cold. What's happened to the pain story? What has changed? I really would like to understand this better."

And Sharon began to rattle on.

"Something clicked. I know it's really up to me now. I was so afraid before. I don't know if you remember that I told you about my grandfather's arthritis. Well, when I was growing up it seems that I was the sick kid. My mother took me to doctors all the time. She kept saying, 'You're just like your grandfather.' Grandpa lived with us. He was always sick. And then he died. The house was crazy so much of the time, and when my mother's boyfriends hung around, inevitably I got sick. I just didn't want to be like my grandpa."

I nodded. "So for a long time you've just felt like there was something basically wrong with you?"

"Yes, that's it. Like I had no control of anything and was somehow destined to be sick and die."

"Ummm."

"I still have pain, but I'm not so afraid now. When my neck starts to hurt sometimes I can even see that I've been working too hard or not getting enough rest or something. I think my body does give me some signals that are meant to help me. I'm really trying to pay attention to my body now. I'm sure this sounds crazy."

"Not at all, Sharon."

"Anyway, it's just a relief to know that the pain makes sense somehow, and to know that I'm not dying from something terrible."

"I think I can see what you mean just a little, Sharon. I'm glad you're finding a way to understand your body and this pain thing. It seems to me that you're also finding some new ways to think about yourself."

"Yes, that's it. I can see that I don't have to be the sick one. I'm starting to see myself as strong and healthy. I think I'm understanding that I can decide the role I want to play. It doesn't have to be dictated by my past–by all that sexual abuse. I think I understood a lot of that in therapy but just hadn't made the connection to what that means in my body."

"Could be," I said.

"And I've even started some volunteer work at the school. I'm busy with my job but I think I'm good with kids and I think I understand some of those kids that live in such dreadful situations. I know about crazy families. A couple of the teachers at the school seem to be pleased with my help."

"Something sure has clicked with you, Sharon."

I realized as we talked that Sharon continued to seem more powerful and I sensed an aliveness in the room.

Two Years Later

I continued to see Sharon occasionally. She continued to have pain but it no longer dominated her life. She became the manager of the housekeeping department at the hotel. She continued to find new ways to understand and be Sharon.

I realized it had been a privilege for me to watch Sharon's change process. Likewise, I realized that I too was struggling with my own change process–trying to find new ways to think about doctors, patients, pain, and healing.

Chapter 2

Impasse and Silent Epidemic

> "Yes, I see you have pain and are upset, Sharon," I responded quickly, relieved that the bricks had stopped flying.
>
> –"Flying Bricks"

In the story in Chapter 1, the extent of Sharon's pain is obvious. The pain has been a focus in her life for many years. In that respect Sharon typifies the person with chronic pain. It seems that Sharon is not alone in this pain business.

Patrick Wall (1991) refers to pain as the silent epidemic and argues that pain is the greatest health problem of our age. Chronic pain syndromes afflict one-third of the American population and together with health care costs and payments for compensation, litigation, and quackery, cost nearly $70 billion annually (Bonica, 1992). These headaches, backaches, muscle pains, joint pains, and menstrual pains probably are also the most mutually frustrating for both patients and doctors.

This probably accounts for the fact that if you watch television or read magazines, inevitably there is some reference to pain. Even though the pain may be the result of tension, worry, poor diet, or excessive exercise, the inevitable response is to reach for the aspirin, tranquilizer, or other analgesic. The message is: don't question the reason for the pain. And yet pain itself is obviously a cause of stress, so we cannot simply conclude that stress is the cause of pain. Furthermore the stories of pain take on many complex variations.

For example:

1. Diane, a 23-year-old woman, experiences headaches. It just so happens she has a history of depression and marital discord. The

doctor thinks the problem is psychiatric. Three months later, after seeing two more physicians, she finally finds a doctor who "listens." She gets the appropriate tests. The results confirm a diagnosis of malignant brain tumor. One year later she dies.

2. Bob, a 42-year-old man, sustains a minor neck injury in a car accident. Three years later the pain persists. He no longer works and his family is in disarray. When he tries to get help, he inevitably feels that he's accused of being a drug user and sinks further into depression.

3. Betty, a 51-year-old woman, experiences persistent bodily pain of a vague nature. Her doctors order endless tests. She has surgeries. Her pain escalates. She and her doctors repeatedly reinforce the notion that her body really is a machine and if the broken part is identified, it could be fixed. Meanwhile, she lives with an alcoholic and abusive man. Neither she nor her doctors have questioned whether marital issues may have some relevance to her pain.

These stories, with their many variations, are daily experiences for physicians and patients. It's not too difficult to see that this is a complex problem for everyone. I don't want to be the doctor to miss the brain tumor. That scares me. I worry about mistakes that harm my patients. I don't want to be incompetent. In a similar fashion, Betty's story of abuse confuses me. I don't think she sees any relationship between abuse and pain. She doesn't talk about it. How can I figure out her problems without increasing her alienation and frustration? And yet I really do want to understand and "help" with the suffering.

When people seek the attention of a doctor, they do so because of a symptom–something is bothering them. They use terms such as "my head hurts," "my feet burn," "my legs ache," etc. Generally the underlying concern is: "What's causing my pain or symptom and can you fix it?" The doctors' training reinforces analytical thinking that is useful in trying to convert the essence of the symptom into some recognizable disease. People expect their symptoms to be a manifestation of a disease and have come to anticipate a diagnosis and cure. Essentially, it's a straightforward task for the doctor to find the "broken" part of the body that has something to do with the symptom, to name the disease, and in turn fix the problem. Unfortunately, not all symptoms fit into concise disease categories. Furthermore, even if they do, it is the person who has the disease, and as such experiences illness and suffering. Needless to say, people aren't just a breast cancer or a heart attack but rather are people who experience these problems. And therein seem to be where doctors and patients together become confused, anxious, and angry, and where they regularly misunderstand each other. Often the meaning of the illness is never explored even if the disease is understood. And if the pain does not translate into body pathology that is readily understood, confusion prevails.

In the story in Chapter 1, I struggle with Sharon about the meaning of the pain in her body. My struggle is to be a competent doctor. I want to diagnose appropriately while at the same time I grapple with the meaning of Sharon's pain. Meanwhile, I also must help Sharon see that there is no easy diagnosis and cure for her. Sharon, however, wants a straightforward diagnosis and expects to be fixed. But in this case it doesn't work that way. Sharon's pain has meaning that transcends a simple explanation. Sharon's chronic pain problem ultimately seems to have some connection to her history of sexual and physical abuse. How this occcurred in Sharon's situation is not clear, but her struggle to express herself and her struggle with her fear about her illness and pain seem connected to the fact that she grew up in an environment where the abuse left her somewhat confused and paralyzed about the meaning and direction of her life. In order for Sharon to heal, which is presumably why she sought my attention in the first place, it became necessary for both of us to struggle with the meaning of her chronic pain. This required moving beyond simplistic answers. This required willingness for both of us to accept uncertainty. It became a challenge to find new approaches.

Paradoxically, in one sense, we all think we know what we mean when we talk about pain. But do we? Even the definition of pain can elude us. The International Association for the Study of Pain (1979, p. 250) defines pain as "an unpleasant sensory and emotional experience associated with actual or potential tissue damage, or described by the patient in terms of such damage." That definition recognizes that pain is a subjective experience. Pain is what we feel. The definition recognizes that pain may exist even in the absence of detectable physical cause. It makes sense that people react to pain based on experience, cultural conditioning, and many other factors.

The differences add up to the suffering the person experiences, and this suffering is a personal experience. It is this personal or subjective part of the pain story that challenges doctors and patients as they work together.

But why and how have doctors and patients reached such misunderstanding around pain problems? Furthermore, how is it that doctors on one hand can offer so much towards the diagnosis and treatment of disease with new and impressive technology, but alternatively seem at such an impasse with understanding the person, their disease and pain, and their suffering?

Physicians have written extensively on this topic. Longhurst (1987) comments: "However, to be a healer, the physician needs a capacity that is beyond the curriculum of the medical school" (p. 38). He argues that the technology of our modern era is no substitute for the healing relationship. To understand this impasse that doctors seem to have with respect to the healing relationship, it seems helpful to glimpse how doctors are trained to think and act. Models are developed to provide a framework for this thinking and acting. A model is an integrated description of a belief system. In their day-to-day work, however, most doctors probably don't think about these models but rather continue to diagnose based on whatever their training emphasized. So when Sharon sought the advice of doctors, there likely was minimal thought by the doctor about models. Rather, the doctors continued to approach the pain problem in the style they had developed from their training. However, to understand the complexity of issues involving women and chronic pain and how women relate to doctors around the topic, some sense of these medical models and how they evolved is necessary.

REFERENCES

Bonica, J.J. (1992). Importance of the problem. In G.M. Aronoff (Ed.). *Evaluation and Treatment of Chronic Pain* (p. xxii). Baltimore: Williams and Wilkins.

International Association for the Study of Pain. (1979). Pain terms: A list with definitions and notes on usage. *Pain* 6:249-252.

Longurst, M.F. (1987). Doctoring: The healing relationship. *Humane Medicine* 3:37-41.

Wall, P.D. and Jones, M. (1991). *Defeating Pain*. New York: Plenum Press.

Chapter 3

Medical Models

> "No, I just think we first need to figure out how we'll work together. What I mean is that you and I will both need to work on understanding this pain stuff and will both need to try a different approach."
>
> –"Flying Bricks"

In Sharon's story, I explain early on in the encounter that we must talk about how we will work together. In some ways this seems redundant. After all, won't we just figure this out as we go along? In most cases doctors and patients do just that. But in this story it is apparent on the first visit that if Sharon and I proceed as she has done with other doctors, we most certainly will end up with the same frustration. For that reason it makes sense for doctors and patients to think together about how we've reached this impasse. This suggests that we look at how doctors think about diagnosis and disease and in turn how they then relate to the patient. For example, have you been to a doctor and told a story of pain, only to wonder whether you and the doctor ultimately are discussing the same issue? Doctors are trained to approach problem solving in a systematic fashion. Understanding how doctors attempt to diagnose and cure pain problems will give insight into the discussion on women and chronic pain. In this chapter I describe the biomedical and biopsychosocial models. I provide historical background to the evolution of these models and conclude with a discussion of the relevance of medical models to patients experiencing pain.

BIOMEDICAL MODEL

Let's observe Dr. X and Patient Y as they interact in a manner consistent with this model.

The Story of Dr. X and Patient Y

Patient Y is a 17-year-old woman who presents in the emergency department with severe abdominal pain. Dr. X takes a careful history. While talking he mentally continues his own analysis of a possible cause for her pain. He realizes there may be something else bothering her as well, but his concern is to first make sure that nothing physical is out of place. This makes sense given the degree of her pain. She answers questions. He examines her body. He does laboratory and radiological tests. He concludes after analyzing all information that her problem is most likely an inflamed appendix. He takes her to the operating room. To his surprise it's not her appendix. She has terrible infection in her fallopian tubes. That's unfortunate, but readily fixed as well. She had denied sexual activity. Therefore, sorting the information had not been easy. Her cultures grew gonorrhea. She readily responds to antibiotic. She is discharged from the hospital. Her discharge summary notes a diagnosis of pelvic inflammatory disease and appendectomy performed. Dr. X informs patient Y of the importance of having her problem followed and advises that her partner be treated. Dr. X is annoyed with himself because he was a little off the diagnosis, but the patient is fixed. The problem was a bug. Antibiotic eradicated the bug. End of story.

Understanding Dr. X

Dr. X typifies the physician who espouses the biomedical model. The biomedical model assumes disease to be fully accounted for by deviations from the norm of measurable biological (somatic) variables (Engel, 1977). It leaves no room within its framework for the social, psychological, and behavioral dimensions of illness. The biomedical model thus embraces both reductionism, the philosophic view that complex phenomena are ultimately derived from a single primary principle, and mind-body dualism, the doctrine that separates the mental from the somatic. A corollary is that whatever is incapable of being explained by physiochemical mechanism should be excluded from the categorization of disease and as such should probably not be the province of physicians or medicine (Medalie, 1990).

How Did This Biomedical Model Develop?

The establishment of medicine as we know it today began in the Middle Ages. The established Christian dogma intermingled with medieval mysticism and exerted an influence on scientific thought well into the nineteenth century. The philosopher Descartes, however, played an important role in the seventeenth century in diminishing the influence of the established Christian church in that he popularized the idea that mind and body are distinct and thus encouraged the emerging scientific approach to disease. Medicine as an institution evolved from this mind-body dualism in response to social needs of the culture.

Descartes viewed the body as a machine and as such saw it as governed by mechanical principles known at the time (Descartes, 1980). Descartes suggested that pain is like a bell-ringing mechanism in a church. He thought that just as a rope is pulled at the bottom of the tower and the bell rings, so pain in the foot travels along nerves scattered throughout the foot and extends from that point all the way to the brain. He thought this produced a certain motion in the brain that produced the feeling of pain. Descartes also attempted to explain pain of a psychological nature by suggesting that a bell could ring in the brain rather than the foot.

Cassell speculates about Descartes' effect on medicine since he formulated the mind-body duality. He comments:

> A cynic may see the Cartesian duality as a tremendously effective solution to the political problem that weighed down the development of science–the Church. By dividing man into mind and body as separate realities and by giving the body over to science and the mind (soul) to philosophy and religion, scientists were able to work without invading the province of God. Whatever the basis of the duality, it is more a part of our

> cultural unconscious than most of us ever realize. In any event, science emerged from the seventeenth century dedicated to a method of thought and having a mission to measure the finite. From that thought mode and mission it has not since deviated. Furthermore, it was in that same historical period that science laid its hand on medicine with a subsequently ever-tightening and jealous grip. (1976, p. 58)

The classification of disease remained largely subjective or descriptive until the germ theory of disease was developed in the late 1800s. This led the way for scientific answers to questions of disease causality. This resulted in the tremendous gains started in the 1930s with the arrival of sulfonamides. Doctors and society entered the age of cure. No one can doubt the magnificence of the drugs, diagnostic tests, and electronic technology. Indeed as we witness the revolution of molecular biology with the mapping of the human genome and tracking the millions of proteins, we are mesmerized. So much promise–so much excitement.

McWhinney (1986) describes how the traditional clinical method used by physicians developed in the nineteenth century along with the biomedical model (1986). The traditional method is strictly objective. The clinician takes a history, conducts a physical exam, and investigates in a prescribed fashion. The aim is to arrive at the pathological diagnosis or be to able to exclude disease. The method does not attempt to understand the meaning of the illness or to place it in the context of the patient's culture.

In spite of tremendous gains for society, this reductionistic approach eventually led to the problems with understanding disease and illness that we see today. Patients and physicians are frustrated. Engel argued for a new model in biomedicine. He suggested that:

> The doctor's task is to account for the dysphoria and the dysfunction which lead individuals to seek medical help, adopt the sick role, and accept the status of patienthood. He must weight the relative contributions of social and psychological as well as of biological factors implicated in the patient's dysphoria and dysfunction as well as in his decision to accept

> or not accept patienthood and with it the responsibility to cooperate in his own health care. (1977, p. 133)

A biopsychosocial model would take all of these factors into account. More recently, Engel comments:

> What advocates of the universality of the biomedical model have failed to appreciate is that, like its 17th century counterpart in classical physics, the biomedical model represents a limiting case the utility of which is in no way diminished as long as its use is restricted to the phenomena for which it was designed. The biomedical model needs no defense, neither with respect to its past accomplishments nor to its future utility, as long as that rule is applied. But to do otherwise is to be unscientific; to advocate doing otherwise is to promote dogma and become antiscientific. To become more fully scientific, medicine requires a paradigm capable of encompassing the human domain. (1992, p. 14)

Whether the biopsychosocial model or other model such as the infomedical model (Foss and Rothenberg, 1987) is the successor to the biomedical model is beyond the scope of this discussion. However, the following comments give insight into the struggle within medicine to embrace the human domain.

BIOPSYCHOSOCIAL MODEL

How might Dr. X (Thomas) interact on the job in the emergency department with Patient Y (Sally) if he espoused the biopsychosocial model?

The Story of Dr. Thomas and Sally

Sally presents in the emergency department with abdominal pain. Dr. Thomas takes a history and asks the usual questions. In addition, he questions her about her social situation. He learns that five months ago her parents separated. She lives with her mother, goes to school, and works. He too concludes after completing the history, physical exam, and laboratory tests that she likely has appendicitis. He also is surprised that the problem turns out to be gonorrhea. He remembers that she specifically told him she wasn't sexually active. After all, with abdominal pain he had to exclude pelvic inflammatory disease, ectopic pregnancy, etc. He suspects Sally may want to talk more. He is concerned. When he talks to her later he carefully explains the diagnosis. He questions her about the discrepancy in the story, while being aware of his desire to be supportive. Eventually Sally talks.

"Someone raped me two months ago," she says. "It happened on my way home from work. I felt frightened. I couldn't talk to my mother. She has too many problems. I'm afraid of the police and hospitals."

She is relieved to finally tell someone the story. He listens. He encourages her. He advises her to see counselors at the sexual assault centre. She is discharged from the hospital. Her discharge summary notes a diagnosis of pelvic inflammatory disease due to gonorrhea, appendectomy, and that she is a sexual assault victim.

Understanding Dr. Thomas

Dr. Thomas embraces the biopsychosocial model. Essentially, in his framework for understanding Sally and her pain he recognized the need to integrate the biological, psychological, and social dimensions of health and disease. In that respect his approach is quite different from that of Dr. X.

MEDICAL MODELS AND THE PATIENT WITH PAIN

So how does this discussion of medical models relate to the patient with pain? Quite simply, people visit doctors because they have symptoms, and symptoms are most frequently expressed as some form of bodily pain or discomfort. And yet it is estimated that in those individuals seen in an outpatient clinic setting, less than one in five symptoms will have an organic explanation (Kroenke, 1992). In other words, the biomedical model provides a useful framework in only 20% of cases. Kroenke concludes that we must continue to dismantle the paradigm of mind-body dualism, the biomedical prejudice that makes a physical explanation for a symptom socially desirable and psychiatric causes stigmatic.

But dismantling this mind-body dualism doesn't seem easy. For example, let's look at irritable bowel syndrome (IBS). This is a puzzling problem. It's a disease that has no clear organic basis, yet many people present to doctors' offices with symptoms of abdominal pain eventually recognized as IBS. The diagnosis is based on a history of continuous or recurrent symptoms for at least three months' duration. Symptoms include: abdominal pain relieved with defecation or associated with a change in the frequency or consistency of stool and an irregular pattern of defecation at least 25% of the time. This is a big problem. Fifteen percent to 20% of people in Western countries suffer from this. Not everyone seeks medical care but 75% to 80% of patients with IBS seen by a physician are female. Interestingly enough the reverse is true in India and Sri Lanka. This problem constitutes 25% to 50% of referrals to gastroenterologists in the United States (Mitchell and Drossman, 1987) and 30% to 60% of referrals to gastroenterologists in Canada (Thompson, 1986). The specialists vary in their approach to the problem.

In a recent issue of the Annals of Internal Medicine, two teams of gastroenterologists discuss IBS and their approaches. Drossman and Thompson (1992) adopt the biopsychosocial approach and emphasize the importance of the therapeutic relationship. Camilleri and Prather (1992) take a methodic approach excluding organic or structural problems before addressing the symptoms. They then focus attention on symptomatic relief with minimal attention to psychosocial issues. This approach would be closer to the biomedical model.

Irritable bowel syndrome obviously frustrates patients along with their doctors. Alternative medicine attracts people with gastrointestinal complaints that doctors call functional to a greater degree than gastrointestinal complaints with an organic cause (Verhoef, Sutherland, and Brkich, 1990). Patients want answers. They want cures. Thompson, in addressing the issues of alternative health care, comments:

> Headaches, low back pain, fibrositis and chronic abdominal pain exist and torment, yet medical science seems powerless to explain or reliably cure. . . . Most patients have conditions for which no technology is of benefit. This reality needs to be made plain to the public and to the media. (1990, pp. 105-6)

The psychiatrists have trouble knowing which model they want to adopt. Hartmann, the 120th president of the American Psychiatric Association, comments:

> Humane values require us, in promoting mental health and fighting mental illness, to be aware of and care for and treat whole people in context and over time: whole biopsychosocial people in context and over time. . . . Reasons for splits and reductionism are many, but in addition to economic pressures, and unbalancing advances in measurable and published research in one or two sector of our field, we may be tempted into reductionism by unacknowledged frustration in a field that seems too big to master, and too bedeviled by outsiders who push us, and sometimes pay us, to simplify. (1992, pp. 1137-38)

It seems like a mess! We've developed impressive technology but have difficulty combining this expertise with the capacity to be healers. This probably has something to do with why Sharon and her doctors kept misunderstanding each other. It's obvious that patient and doctor alike often want easy answers and cures. We're all of us somehow in this together. It seems that the fascination with reductionism and the tendency in the culture to reinforce the virtues of the biomedical model keep all of us crippled. Furthermore, the strictly objective stance of the physician that has developed along with the biomedical model simply doesn't want to disappear. After all, isn't it easier to be an objective, rational, detached, scientific physician than a physician who really has to get in there with all those mucky emotional responses? Doctors, and in many cases patients, are uncomfortable with complexity and the messiness of emotional responses. It seems it's just too frustrating to shift into behavior more consistent with the biopsychosocial model.

But in addition to how doctors perceive that they solve problems is the question of what we mean about pain. In order to discuss chronic pain that women experience we need a sense of how we share information about pain. This requires that we differentiate between acute and chronic pain and begin to address the meaning of pain problems. In Chapter 4, I discuss acute pain and the way chronic pain needs to be differentiated from acute pain.

REFERENCES

Camilleri, M. and Prather, C.M. (1992). The irritable bowel syndrome: mechanisms and a practical approach to management. *Ann Intern Med* 116:1001-1008.

Cassell, E.J. (1976). *The Healer's Art.* Cambridge, MA: MIT Press.

Descartes, R. (1980). *Discourse on Method and Meditations on First Philosophy* (Original work published 1637/1641). Indianapolis:Hackett Publishing.

Drossman, D.A. and Thompson, W.G. (1992). The irritable bowel syndrome: review and a graduated multicomponent treatment approach. *Ann Intern Med* 116:1009-1016.

Engel, G.L. (1977). The need for a new model: a challenge for biomedicine. *Science* 196:129-136.

_______ . (1992). How much longer must medicine's science be bound by a seventeenth century world view? *Psychother Psychosom* 57:3-16.

Foss, L. and Rothenberg, K. (1987). *The Second Medical Revolution. From Biomedicine to Infomedicine.* Boston: Shambhala, New Science Library.

Hartmann, L. (1992). Presidential address: reflections on humane values and biopsychosocial integration. *Am J Psychiatry* 149:1135-1141.

Kroenke, K. (1992). Symptoms in medical patients: an untended field. *Am J Med* 92(suppl 1A):1A-3S-1A-6S.

McWhinney, I.R. (1986). Are we on the brink of a major transformation of clinical method? *Can Med Assoc J* 135:873-878.

Medalie, J.H. (1990). Angina pectoris: a validation of the biopsychosocial model. *J Fam Pract* 30:273-280.

Mitchell, C.M. and Drossman, D.A. (1987). Survey of the AGA membership relating to patients with functional gastrointestinal disorders (Letter). *Gastroenterology* 92:1282-1284.

Thompson, W.G. (1986). Irritable bowel syndrome: prevalence, prognosis and consequences (E). *Can Med Assoc J* 134:111-113.

_______ . (1990). Alternatives to medicine. *Can Med Assoc J* 142:105-106.

Verhoef, M.J., Sutherland, L.R., and Brkich, L. (1990). Use of alternative medicine by patients attending a gastroenterology clinic. *Can Med Assoc J* 142:121-125.

Chapter 4

Acute Pain and Chronic Pain

> "I hurt mostly in my neck and upper back. Sometimes I get headaches. I think I hurt most of the time but some days are worse than others. The pain never leaves."
>
> –"Flying Bricks"

In order to further explore issues related to women and chronic pain, it is important to understand how we think and talk about pain. For instance, Sharon and I used many words about the pain–hurt, worse, better, headaches, pain stuff, hurt so much, etc. However, it is likely that as we shared information we often differed even about the meaning of these simple words. In this chapter, I discuss acute pain, the mechanisms of pain, and the ways chronic pain differs from acute pain.

THE STORY OF ACUTE PAIN

"Ouch, It Hurts"

On a warm summer day a few years ago, I hiked one of the wonderful trails in the Canadian Rockies. My backpack as usual seemed too heavy, but I persisted. I noticed white clouds floating over the rocks. I breathed in the clear mountain air. I pondered deeply as I walked along. Mostly I felt alive.

And then we came to the stream. My track record with streams wasn't great. Falling off logs and slipping on stones seemed my forte. This stream looked gentle. I felt relieved. Carefully, I negotiated the wet rocks. It happened. My hand dug into the bottom of the creek bed. My body plopped into the water. Mountain water is incredibly cold. I quickly got up and reached the other side. Initially I felt annoyed. That concern quickly subsided as I realized I felt nauseated, faint, and unwell. I stretched out on the ground. My forehead became cold and clammy. Eventually, I realized that my finger hurt. I noticed the bruising. The painful sensation in my finger persisted.

I gradually recovered and continued to hike. I chose to ignore the persisting pain and the swollen finger. Two days later, I reluctantly consulted a physician. Along with help from the X-ray department, the physician diagnosed a broken finger.

UNDERSTANDING ACUTE PAIN

Generally, it's not too difficult to appreciate an experience of acute pain. Acute pain is of recent onset. There is tissue damage and the pain diminishes as the healing occurs. Over 90% of people with these injuries will recover in eight weeks. The injuries are accompanied by psychological reactions such as simple fright and anxiety. The body responds with autonomic changes that may include increased heart rate, changes in blood pressure, sweating hands, etc., the sort of thing I experienced at the edge of the stream. The duration of the acute pain can usually be predicted by the physician when the cause of the pain is known. In a very real way both doctors and patients are comfortable with the acute pain problem because it fits the biomedical model to a large degree.

It would be easier to understand pain if the degree of injured tissue was simply directly related to the sensation of pain. Scientific research has shown that the injury and pain business are very complex. Many opinions and many ideas.

THINKING ABOUT ACUTE AND CHRONIC PAIN SIMULTANEOUSLY

In an attempt to understand chronic pain, the focus of this book, it is necessary to briefly look at pain models because chronic pain is different from acute pain. Chronic pain outlasts the recognized natural stimulus. It becomes separate from the evidences of nociception. Nociception is defined as a response that occurs specifically to potentially tissue-damaging stimulation. Nociception is not the same as pain perception. Pain perception involves our minds and emotions along with physical sensations.

That seems to be where patients and doctors get stuck. We keep wanting to think about all pain as if it were acute pain. We keep thinking about pain as tissue injury. When diagnostic tests don't reveal damaged anatomy, patients think: (1) the doctor believes it's all in my head; or (2) that's an incompetent doctor because I'm in pain and it can't be found or fixed. Doctors in turn think: (1) the problem isn't real and I don't need to "solve" it; or (2) the pain is psychogenic–how do I get them to a psychiatrist?

Certainly that seems to be where Sharon and her doctors were stuck. When the doctors couldn't find the damaged anatomy, Sharon inevitably felt "they don't believe it hurts." Doctors in turn obviously felt frustrated: "What's really wrong with this woman and why does she hurt if the tests are all normal?" To address this further let's look at how doctors presently understand pain.

MECHANISMS OF PAIN

Standard textbooks describing mechanisms of pain are filled with phrases like: neurons of the substangia gelatinosa, presynaptic inhibition, dorsal root potential, dendrites of islet cells and primary afferent somatosensory. A detailed discussion at that level would be distracting. Attempts to simplify will be inaccurate, but for this discussion I'll aim for the essence of the topic.

Our bodies contain receptors that are sensitive to heat, pressure, cold, etc. When these receptors are stimulated by hockey sticks, hot coffee, or ice cubes they produce electrical charges that travel along nerve fibers through the spinal cord to the brain. How we feel and experience the pain, as a result of the stimulation, is a topic of continued debate. Models of pain evolved over the first part of this century, culminating in the gate control theory described by Melzack and Wall (1965). Essentially, interactions between the different types of nerve fibers were thought to open or shut a gate, thereby increasing or decreasing the intensity of the pain message. This theory continues to be revised with increasing complexity (Hoffert, 1992). Pain perception is influenced by messages moving up to the brain as well as descending messages from the brain that can block or change ascending messages. This draws attention to the importance of considering psychological factors in pain perception and tolerance.

Since the publication of the gate-control theory, changes in pain management have occurred. The use of destructive neurosurgical techniques has declined while stimulation analgesia and the use of spinal opioids has received attention. Many experts point to the benefits of psychological assessment in the management of chronic pain (Macrae, Davies, and Crombie, 1992). However, because pain is the person's private experience, chronic pain problems have continued to perplex and frustrate patient and physician alike.

What does Sharon really mean when she says the pain never leaves. Certainly there must be a moment here or there when she is pain-free. Let's take a closer look at chronic pain.

THE STORY OF CHRONIC PAIN

"But It Still Hurts"

Let's look at another day in the Canadian Rockies. This time–the ski slope. I pride myself in my skill in this area. I ski fast and love the physical sensation of speed. Normally all goes well. On this particular day the light on the slope was flat. That means there's no sunshine peeking through the thick layer of clouds. Consequently, even if the slope has many bumps, there can be a perception of no bumps. I skied fast down the slope, counting on my feet to give messages to my brain about the bumps so that I could adjust knees, upper body, etc. It didn't work. As I planted my nose squarely on the hill in front of and below me, I extended my neck in a horrible fashion. Not too surprisingly, I suffered a neck injury.

This time I took immediate advantage of the health care facilities. I attended physiotherapy faithfully. Six months later my neck still hurt. I couldn't work at my usual pace. Even attempts to play the piano resulted in severe pain. Life began to revolve around the painful neck. I no longer had an acute problem. The chronic neck pain persisted even with medical treatment and the passage of time.

UNDERSTANDING CHRONIC PAIN

Chronic pain is generally defined as the occurrence of daily pain over an extended period of time–usually six months or longer. The pain outlasts the recognized stimulus. Chronic pain problems represent a spectrum of problems. On one hand, we speak of chronic pain in association with chronic illness such as cancer and arthritis. These concerns are different from chronic pain following an obvious injury. Low back pain is the chronic pain problem that creates endless dilemmas in the work force. Here, the pain persists long after the injury occurred, and the degree of pain generally seems out of proportion to the extent of the injury. On the other hand are chronic pain problems in which a physical injury has never been apparent. Irritable bowel syndrome, as discussed in Chapter 3, would be an example of this type of chronic pain.

As would be expected, most people experiencing chronic pain problems, irrespective of the type of chronic problem, eventually also endure family disturbance, altered life-style, and economic problems. These issues become major problems in themselves. Not too surprisingly, the chronic pain becomes associated with depression and other emotional distress.

TREATMENT OF CHRONIC PAIN

It's no mystery that doctors and patients are equally challenged when it comes to treating chronic pain sufferers. Specialized pain treatment centers have emerged in many communities; however, the diversity of these centers is readily acknowledged (Csordas and Clark, 1992). Baszanger (1992), studying two centers specializing in the treatment of chronic pain patients explored the very different approaches that exist with chronic pain management. He suggests that the management of chronic pain is taking shape around two very different poles. On one extreme, the aim is to cure pain by means ranging from drugs and the simplest physical methods to more sophisticated neurosurgical techniques. The other approach is the control of pain, which resorts to cognitive and behavioral techniques along with drugs and physical therapy. The cognitive-behavioral approach focuses not only on behavior, but also on cognitive (perceptive) and affective (emotional) components of the pain experience (Keefe and Burnett, 1992). The behavioral approach aims to modify maladaptive pain behaviors by analyzing and changing the social and environmental contingencies. These approaches emphasize the patient's participation in learning management techniques. The aim is to minimize pain as opposed to curing the pain.

Another area of growing clinical interest and research concerns the relationship between family functioning and the individual suffering from chronic, intractable pain. Pain may serve some purpose, consciously or otherwise in organizing the family. This family systems orientation becomes another model for understanding pain (Margolis et al., 1991). The psychological management of chronic pain has seen many different approaches (Philips, 1988; Miller, 1993).

As would be expected, research in the chronic pain area is plagued with many problems due to the nature of the problem itself. In addition, most studies on chronic pain patients have relied on samples of low back pain patients, which of course represents only one problem. Determining outcome is difficult. Turk and Rudy (1991) found that 30% to 60% of chronic pain patients treated successfully eventually relapsed. In a recent review of outcome studies, Turk, Rudy, and Sorkin (1993) point out that investigators simply do not agree about how patient improvement should be determined. Again, the elusive, subjective nature of pain presents problems.

Most patients, however, are not treated at pain clinics. Individual physicians vary greatly in their approach to and understanding of chronic pain problems. Goldman (1991) reports that ignorance of chronic pain on the part of the medical profession is a major issue. Medical schools give low priority to training in chronic-pain management, and research in this area doesn't attract the attention of the more technical specialties. A major challenge, as seen by Macrae,

Davies and Crombie (1992), is changing doctors' perception of pain and methods of treatment, not just amongst pain clinicians, but in the wider medical community.

As I have suggested, understanding and treating chronic pain is an issue for everyone. Doctors and patients struggle with the complexity of the problems and rarely find simplistic answers. But do women experiencing chronic pain have other concerns? Most discussion on chronic pain, whether in textbooks, at continuing medical education courses, or in the medical literature, rarely includes gender issues. This assumes that men and women have similar concerns around chronic pain. And yet, women are the predominant sufferers of chronic pain in which obvious physical injury or obvious organic pathology is absent. Since this is the case, do we not need to question why women are prone to particular types of chronic pain problems? Furthermore, is it possible to fully discuss chronic pain problems that women experience without also making an attempt to see how our current medical scientific ideas are infused by cultural assumptions? In Chapter 5, I take a closer look at chronic pain problems women experience and in Chapter 6 address questions of gender and medical culture.

REFERENCES

Baszanger, I. (1992). Deciphering chronic pain. *Sociology of Health and Illness* 14:181-215.

Csordas, T.J. and Clark, J.A. (1992). Ends of the line: diversity among chronic pain centers. *Soc Sci Med* 34:383-393.

Goldman, B. (1991). Chronic-pain patients must cope with chronic lack of physician understanding. *Can Med Assoc J* 144:1492-1497.

Hoffert, M.J. (1992). The neurophysiology of pain. In: G.M. Aronoff, (Ed.), *Evaluation and Treatment of Chronic Pain* (pp.10-25). Philadelphia: Williams and Wilkins.

Keefe, F.J. and Burnett, R. (1992). Behavioral and cognitive-behavioral approaches to chronic pain: recent advances and future directions. *J Consult Clin Psychol* 60:528-536.

Macrae, W.A., Davies, H.T.O., and Crombie, I.K. (1992). Pain: paradigms and treatments. *Pain* 49:289-291.

Margolis, R.B., Merkel, W.T., Tait, R.C., and Richardson, W. (1991). Evaluating patients with chronic pain and their families. *Can Fam Physician* 37:429-435.

Melzack, R. and Wall, P.D. (1965). Pain mechanisms: a new theory. *Science* 150:971-979.

Miller, L. (1993). Psychotherapeutic approaches to chronic pain. *Psychotherapy* 30:115-124.

Philips, H.C. (1988). *The Psychological Management of Chronic Pain.* New York: Springer.

Turk, D.C. and Rudy, R.E. (1991). Neglected topics in the treatment of chronic pain patients: relapse, noncompliance, and adherence enhancement. *Pain* 44:5-28.

Turk, D.C., Rudy, T.E., and Sorkin, B.A. (1993). Neglected topics in chronic pain treatment outcome studies: determination of success. *Pain* 53:3-16.

Chapter 5

Women and Elusive Pain

"Well, I'm not completely sure yet but from your story, check up, and the tests you've had you look like you have fibromyalgia. That's just a fancy name for a type of pain problem that tends to affect your back, neck, and other parts of your body. People have these tender points just like you do. The frustrating thing is that the problem isn't understood very well. There are no clear tests to diagnose the problem and no easy solutions."

–"Flying Bricks"

In Sharon's story, I explain to her that her pain has a label but that the problem–fibromyalgia–is not well understood. I explain that there are no simple tests or easy solutions. Pain problems with no readily identified organic explanations are the problems that plague doctors and patients alike. These problems cannot be understood within the biomedical model. Alternatively, pain associated with chronic disease such as cancer or heart disease is not perplexing. There is a biologic basis for the pain. Pain that is associated with an injury can become distressing when the pain does not resolve as expected, but even with these pain problems the pain story has meaning that can be discussed and understood in some sense.

Men and women both suffer chronic pain problems, but why are women the predominant sufferers of pain problems where no biologic problem is readily identified? Let's take a quick look at some of these chronic pain problems and the evidence that these problems are major issues for women. The problems discussed are not meant to be an exhaustive summary, but rather to focus on more common chronic pain problems prevalent to women.

Irritable bowel syndrome (discussed in Chapter 3) is a disorder characterized by abdominal pain and discomfort. The problem occurs in men and women, but 75% to 80% of patients seen by consultants in North America are women. This problem accounts for 25% to 50% of referrals to gastroenterologists in the United States and 30% to 60% of referrals to gastroenerologists in Canada. Obviously a big problem. This problem is diagnosed solely on history and the exclusion of other problems. There is no laboratory test or radiologic examination to make the diagnosis and no clear understanding of pathology in the gastrointestinal track to account for the problem.

Fibromyalgia is another common problem seen by physicians. This disorder is characterized by tender spots on the body that are extremely painful to touch. Fibromyalgia occurs ten times more often in women than in men (Goldenberg, 1992). It occurs most frequently between ages 25 and 50. Again, the diagnosis of fibromyalgia is based on the history and physical examination, rather than diagnositic tests that demonstrate organic pathology. In addition, 40% to 60% of people with fibromyalgia have irritable bowel syndrome (IBS). People with both IBS and fibromyalgia have a high incidence of chronic headache and migraines (Watson et al., 1978).

Chronic pelvic pain is another problem commonly occurring with or confused with IBS. Chronic pelvic pain accounts for 10% of outpatient gynecologic consultations and is the indication for up to 25% of diagnostic laparoscopies (Reiter and Gambone, 1989). Multiple studies have shown that chronic pelvic pain is often unrelated to demonstrable organic pathology.

In a recent editorial on gender and pain, Ruda (1993) notes that there are many examples of pain problems that disproportionately affect women. Headache and rheumatoid arthritis are often cited. Lipton et al. (1993) found that on data collected as part of the 1989 National Health Interview Survey, women were consistently higher than men for all reported types of orofacial pain. Women had nearly twice the rate of jaw joint pain than men, and more than twice the rate for face pain.

Somatoform pain disorder, a problem characterized by preoccupation with pain in the absence of adequate physical findings, is diagnosed almost twice as frequently in females as in males (Diagnostic and Statistical Manual of Mental Disorders-III-R, Third Edition, Revised, 1987). Another problem experienced almost exclusively by women and described in the psychiatric literature is somatization disorder. The diagnosis for this problem depends on recognizing a long-standing pattern of seeking medical intervention for vague, multisystemic symptoms without clear physical cause. This disorder was initially defined as a form of hysteria. It may be argued that this is not really a pain problem but the overlap is obvious. Many of the symptoms that women who are diagnosed with somatization disorder describe, will be descriptions of pain.

Beyond the obvious physical component of the pain problems just mentioned, there is a recognition that these problems are generally associated with some degree of mental distress, commonly depression and anxiety. Depression is consistently diagnosed more frequently in women than in men (Notman, 1989).

The obvious comments are: "so, women have lots of pain with little evidence of organic pathology," "so, women are socialized to seek help more than men," "so, it's not surprising that doctors may tend to dismiss women's stories of pain," "these women really aren't diseased," "there's nothing wrong with them," "so, women are the more passive, dependent sex," etc. The traditional medical approach seems permeated with this overtone.

Is there another way to look at this woman-pain issue?

ANOTHER PERSPECTIVE ON WOMEN AND CHRONIC PAIN

I believe that addressing this question requires us to determine whether the ideas generated are the essence of "Hismedicine" or alternately "Hermedicine"–a form of medicine in which the female experience is validated and understood within the context of the culture.

To explore that idea let's take a brief look at somatization disorder, a problem characterized by multiple vague complaints but no organic disorder. "Hismedicine" has tended to view somatization disorder from one perspective. In a recent article, Quill (1985) referred to somatization disorder as one of medicine's blind spots. In the paper, Quill outlines an interesting story that is typical for this disorder. He reports the case of a 74-year-old woman, who over the course of a short time saw a neurologist, a cardiologist, a gastroenterologist, and a pulmonologist. Her evaluation included many tests. Understanding the following list of tests is not necessary, but the extent of the investigation is impressive. She received the following diagnostic tests: two computed tomographic scans of the head, two electroencephalograms, nerve conduction studies, a muscle biopsy, an echocardiogram, a cardiac catherization, a stress-thallium test, a barium enema, two endoscopies, two colonoscopies, pulmonary function tests, and two ventilation-perfusion scans. Her more remote history showed over 30 surgeries and she had carried over 50 separate medical diagnoses. He notes that she described having had a "hard life," including two siblings who had died violent deaths, a mother who had died painfully of bowel carcinoma, and a long marriage to an alcoholic husband who had physically abused her. She had worked hard since childhood, the only respite being periods when she was ill.

He suggests that for the patient with a somatization disorder, symptoms and illness become a way of life. They become a form of communication, a means of expressing emotions, and a way of controlling the environment. He concludes that to be therapeutic to a somatizing patient, the physician must scale down his expectations of himself and his belief in the power of biotechnical medicine. In addition, Quill comments that highly skilled physicians repeatedly fail to recognize patients with somatization disorders.

But how might "Hermedicine" view this problem? Is it reasonable to refer to these physicians as highly skilled? Alternatively, could we not ask why the male-dominated medical profession is so obsessed with the power of biotechnical medicine and so unable to understand the need to comfort the suffering person? Why have physicians been so reluctant to move beyond the biomedical model? Why do physicians repeatedly address all pain problems as if they were acute pain problems? Why is it not a reasonable expectation that doctors would attempt to explore the meaning of pain with their patients? Does the obsessive focus on diagnostic tests that physicians manifest become a problem that needs a diagnostic label?

But are there other questions to ask? Are we blinded in other ways? What is it about our culture that woman regularly resort to controlling their environment through the expression of physical pain? What did it mean for the woman in the story to have a "hard life"? What is the meaning of the physically abusive husband in terms of her health? What about the culture in which spousal abuse is so common? How often does chronic pain in women represent a form of communication, or an attempt to be heard? Are women silenced in the doctor's office? What about the medical culture?

In a discussion of the limits of reductionism and the Cartesian paradigms, Onnis comments:

> If a sick body is reduced to a "natural sign" and deprived of meaning–if a sick body can only be "described," not "interpreted"–then it can offer no clues that permit the doctor to understand and cure the disorder. . . . The attitude of detached neutrality, which is often taken in the name of so-called scientific objectivity, limits the doctor's contact with the patient to the examination and treatment of the organic disorder. The doctor therefore tends, *de facto*, to *deny the relationship* with the patient, which puts the doctor in an untenable, paradoxical situation. Because it is impossible *not* to communicate, the doctor inevitably transmits a message to the patient: "You exist only as a sick body." And this message is transmitted with all the authority of a technically competent person speaking in the name of science. That is why the patient ends up adapting himself or herself to this authority and message, to the extent that, in the end, it is the patient who presents his or her body to the doctor as an object to be repaired, thereby distancing the doctor from the sense of suffering the patient is experiencing. (1993, pp. 140, 143)

It's not too difficult to understand how the woman in the case report ended up with all the investigation, but ultimately minimal sense of meaning, of her pain. No wonder women with chronic pain problems and no organic pathology often are frustrated along with their doctors. The traditional medical approach within the framework of the biomedical model quite simply does not allow for the meaning of symptoms to emerge. In the next chapter, I take a closer look at the medical culture and what this means for women with chronic pain.

REFERENCES

Goldenberg, D.L. (1992). Controversies in fibromyalgia and myofascial pain syndrome. In G.M. Aronoff (Ed.), *Evaluation and Treatment of Chronic Pain* (pp. 165-175). Baltimore: Williams and Wilkins.

Lipton, J.A., Ship, J.A., and Larach-Robinson, D. (1993). Estimated prevalence and distribution of reported orofacial pain in the United States. *JADA* 124:115-121.

Notman, M.T. (1989). Depression in women. In B.L. Parry (Ed.). *Psychiatr Clin North Am* 12:221-230.

Onnis, L. (1993). Psychosomatic medicine: toward a new epistemology. *Fam Syst Med* 11:137-148.

Quill, T.E. (1985). Somatization disorder. *JAMA* 254:3075-3079.

Reiter, R.C. and Gambone, J.C. (1989). Demographic and historical variable in women with idiopathic chronic pelvic pain. *Obstet Gynecol* 75:428-432.

Ruda, M.A. (1993). Gender and pain. *Pain* 53:1-2.

Watson, W.C., Sullivan, S.N., Corke, M., and Rush, D. (1978). Globus and headache: common symptoms of the irritable bowel syndrome. *Can Med Assoc J* 118:387-388.

Chapter 6

Medical Culture

> "But I think maybe the abuse is part of all of this pain stuff. You know, there has been so much pain. I always wondered about things but doctors never asked so I thought it couldn't be connected. And I have always been so afraid–afraid that there's something terribly wrong with my body–afraid that everyone could see what's wrong with me."
>
> –"Flying Bricks"

In the story in Chapter 1, I commented that I felt stunned when Sharon suggested that doctors aren't interested in messy stuff (referring to the abuse history). And yet, in all honesty, certainly I wasn't stunned. Rather, I likely felt shock that I was beginning to have a sense of Sharon's story that I had previously rarely explored with patients in my practice. Most likely, I also felt defensive. After all, we doctor's do care about you–how can you suggest we aren't interested, etc.?

Ultimately, I questioned: How did I, as a physician, overlook, exclude, and fail to understand the degree to which women with chronic pain often have histories of abuse? In time, I began to have glimpses of the ways the dominant medical cultural view often diminishes women's experiences and why this is of particular concern for women who experience chronic pain problems.

In the previous chapters I discussed medical models and how we discuss and understand pain. I made no reference to culture or gender. Burkett argues that the biopsychosocial model also has limitations. He notes that this model tends to treat culture as though it were a tangential characteristic of the human animal. He comments:

> In failing to fully acknowledge how rooted the healer and patient alike are in specific cultural systems, the biopsychosocial model–like much cross-cultural medicine–understates the importance of the negotiation between alternative belief systems that occurs in the medical encounter. (1991, p. 289)

And generally, unless we are consciously trying to increase our awareness about these issues, we tend to think and work with minimal sense of our own cultural orientation. For example, I perceived myself as a competent doctor that cared. I had minimal awareness of how my training reinforced my sense of power and superior knowledge, and how this in turn limited my interaction with patients and other health professionals. Or, how I regularly limited my patient's stories and all too often "judged" women such as Sharon, who experienced chronic pain problems, as somehow inferior or having problems that were less important than, for example, heart disease or cancer.

The topic of culture and gender in medicine is complex. Howard Stein, in his book titled *American Medicine as Culture*, argues that the very organization and practice of medicine are themselves cultural. He comments:

> The official and officially taught medical worldview consists of (1) the "basic sciences": anatomy, physiology, biochemistry, microbiology, pathology; (2) the belief that medical science is and should be based upon rational, scientific, dispassionate, objective, professional judgment; (3) the belief that disease and its attendant suffering are ultimately to be understood in terms of pathological entities, organic in nature, and that treatment optimally consists of a technological procedure or intervention that results in a cure; (4) the belief that medical knowledge and skills are best organized by creating specialties around "organ systems." This official ethos is only the surface or manifest part of a complex cultural picture. I argue that for practitioners and teachers, the biomedical ethos often functions less as scientific reality testing than as an intricate per-

> sonal, group, institutional, and cultural defense against the experience of vulnerability, fragility, infirmity, aggression, sexual desire, passivity, and death–in short, abhorred qualities or characteristics associated with patienthood. (1990, p. xiv)

It can be difficult, as a physician, to begin to see that your approach has as much to do with protecting you as with trying to diagnose and cure your patients. As Sharon and other women shared their stories with me, together we moved away from an objective stance. I became aware of my own struggles to value the subjective world of my patients and at the same time begin to value my subjective experience. As I moved into dialogue with women around their abuse and pain experiences, I increasingly became aware of my own vulnerability and fragility. I sensed I began to open to the notion that my stance as an objective, rational, scientific physician protected me as much as it functioned to project the notion of the expert professional. Likewise, I began to form a different perspective around Sharon's comment that "doctors aren't interested in messy stuff." I began to see that this statement had something to do with Sharon, but also had a great deal to do with how the medical profession has developed in this culture.

The male doctor as expert and scientist did not emerge in North America without struggle. Ehrenreich and English in telling the story of the rise of the experts comment:

> The story of the rise of the psychomedical experts–the doctors, the psychologists, and sundry related professional–might be told as an allegory of science versus superstition: on the one side, the clear-headed, masculine spirit of science; on the other side, a dark morass of female superstition, old wives' tales, rumors preserved as fact. In this allegorical version, the triumph of science was as inevitable as human progress or natural evolution: the experts triumphed because they were right. (1978, p. 33)

They go on to state that the real story is not so simple, and the outcome not so clearly "progressive." The transformation of regular medicine into "scientific medicine" is indeed a story told from many different perspectives depending on the view you choose. But the result was the emergence in the twentieth century of a male-dominated system of medicine–a system in which the scientist and his objective world were elevated and transformed. In a sense, medical science took on a sacred quality.

There is a negative side, however, to the emergence of this sacred medical science. Rich notes:

> The dominant male culture, in separating man as knower from both woman and from nature as the objects of knowledge, evolved certain intellectual polarities which still have the power to blind our imagination. Any deviance from a quality valued by that culture can be dismissed as negative: where "rationality" is posited as sanity, legitimate method, "real thinking," and alternative, intuitive, supersensory, or poetic knowledge are labelled "irrational." . . . Moreover, the "rational" relegated to its opposite term all that it refuses to deal with, and thus ends by assuming itself to be purified of the nonrational, rather than searching to identify and assimilate its own surreal or nonlinear elements. This single error may have mutilated patriarchal thinking–especially scientific and philosophic thinking–more than we yet understand. (1976, p. 62)

The degree to which technology has been valued in the medical culture is easy to see. Sharon sensed that "doctors aren't interested in messy stuff." This observation most certainly wasn't just about Sharon. Sharon repeatedly saw doctors where it's reasonable to conclude that the doctors perceived themselves as the knower and that Sharon too perceived this and in no sense viewed herself as the knowledgeable one. There was no sense of both doctor and patient together trying to understand the pain problem. The notion of the doctor as the powerful one who labels problems is ingrained in the culture. This has been particularly damaging for women patients. Whether at the personal level or at the larger social level women repeatedly receive messages that devalue their personal knowledge.

What has this meant for women in doctor's offices? Most certainly, it has meant that given the degree to which the male-dominated medical culture plays in determining the labeling of "disease," the voice of the individual woman in the doctor's office may be expected to be silenced. Her opinions, her knowledge, her ideas, may not be valued.

In discussing the role of the medical culture in the labeling of disease, Abbey and Garfinkel (1991) point out the similarities between neurasthenia (a disorder characterized by abnormal fatigability) in the nineteenth century and chronic fatigue syndrome today. Each developed in an era characterized by public concern about the fast pace of life and the changing role of women. Showalter (1985) noted that physicians in the late nineteenth century made explicit links between women's ambition and the upsurge in three diseases that occurred predominantly among females–neurasthenia, hysteria, and anorexia nervosa. Women's expression of pain must be understood within this male-dominated culture.

What has it meant for women when personal experiences are devalued, when subjective information is lost, and when ultimately consulting with a physician means giving the information he wants, information that he can understand within his framework of disease? What has it meant when physical, sexual, and emotional abuse that women experience has been locked behind closed doors and has not been seen to be part of disease? What has it meant when women in pain are not heard because the system keeps the door shut?

Hamilton, in discussing the need for humanistic change in women's health care research and practice, comments:

> The dominant perspective within medicine as a whole involves an implicit theory, biological primacy, which operates, cognitively, as extra baggage, creating problems in offering humane health care in general and, more so, in understanding and addressing women's health needs in particular. . . . The feminist critique embodies a substantial challenge to traditional power relationships in the medical profession, and it challenges the biomedical model in and of itself. The biomedical model devalues emotional aspects of healing. (1993, p. 51)

In thinking about Sharon and other women who have shared their stories and how I related to them, I ask myself: Can I really understand the degree to which I repeatedly experienced the ways that man as opposed to woman is rational knower in this culture and how this inevitably left me unable to hear women or to value my own intuitive knowledge? The comment, "Nellie, you're a physician–think like a man not like a woman," a comment told as a joke, no longer seems funny. Certainly, I learned to be a "male physician." I learned to value the rational and objective world. I learned to devalue subjective knowledge. I learned to devalue personal knowledge. It no longer seems such a mystery that women such as Sharon repeatedly felt "not heard" in the doctor's office and repeatedly hoped the doctor and knower would fix them.

REFERENCES

Abbey, S.E. and Garfinkel, P.E. (1991). Neurasthenia and chronic fatigue syndrome: the role of culture in the making of a diagnosis. *Am J Psychiatry* 148:1638-1646.

Burkett, G.L. (1991). Culture, illness, and the biopsychosocial model. *Fam Med* 23:287-291.

Ehrenreich, B. and English, D. (1978). *For Her Own Good.* New York: Doubleday.

Hamilton, J.A. (1993). Feminist theory and health psychology: tools for an egalitarian, woman-centered approach to women's health. *J Women's Health* 2:49-54.

Rich, A. (1976). *Of Woman Born.* New York: W.W. Norton.

Showalter, E. (1985). *The Female Malady: Women, Madness and English Culture, 1830-1980.* New York: Pantheon Books.

Stein, H.F. (1990). *American Medicine as Culture.* Boulder: Westview Press.

Chapter 7

The Association Between Chronic Pain and Abuse

> "Sharon, this sounds painful," I responded quickly, "but I think there is a connection and I've heard so many women say this–this thing about being afraid that there is something terribly wrong with their body as a result of the abuse."
>
> –"Flying Bricks"

The last decade has seen an increasing interest in the topic of violence as a health issue. Stories of physical and sexual abuse emerge from all ethnic and socioeconomic groups. The obvious physical and psychological trauma is not difficult to imagine. The medical literature on the correlation between sexual and/or physical abuse and psychiatric illness is extensive. Along with this literature, however, are a few reports that I think are of particular interest in a discussion of women and chronic pain.

Domino and Haber (1987), reporting from a multidisciplinary pain center, found that of their sample of 30 women with headaches, 66% had experienced prior physical and/or sexual abuse. These women reported a significantly greater number of surgical procedures than the nonabused women.

Drossman et al. (1990), in studying women with functional and organic gastrointestinal disorders found that a history of sexual and physical abuse was a frequent although hidden experience in women seen in a referral-based gastroenterology practice. Patients with functional disorders (IBS, the most frequent diagnosis in this group) were more likely than those with organic disease diagnoses to report a history of forced intercourse and frequent physical abuse, chronic or recurrent abdominal pain, and more lifetime surgeries. Abused patients were more likely than nonabused patients to report pelvic pain, multiple somatic symptoms, and more lifetime surgeries. Similarly, Walker et al. (1993), compared patients with inflammatory bowel disease (ulcerative colitis or Crohn's disease, both problems with clearly defined biologic etiology) to those with irritable bowel syndrome and found that patients with irritable bowel syndrome had a significantly higher rate of severe lifetime sexual trauma (32% versus 0%), severe childhood sexual abuse (11% versus 0%), and any lifetime sexual victimization (54% versus 5%), than those patients with inflammatory bowel disease.

Several reports indicate an association between chronic pelvic pain and a history of sexual and/or physical abuse. Rapkin et al. (1990) reported that the pernicious nature of abuse, whether physical or sexual, may promote the chronicity of pelvic pain. In a study of 36 chronic pelvic pain patients, Toomey et al. (1993) found that the 19 women reporting abuse experienced less perceived life control, greater punishing responses to pain, and higher levels of somatization and global distress than the nonabused group. Harrop-Griffiths et al. (1988) found that women with chronic pelvic pain had experienced significantly more childhood and adult sexual abuse than had controls. Reiter found that previous sexual abuse was a significant predisposing risk for women experiencing chronic pelvic pain problems not associated with organic pathology (1991).

In a study comparing women with somatization disorder and women with affective (mood) disorder, Morrison (1989) found that the two groups reported similar sexual experiences except that significantly more women with somatization disorder had been molested as children. In a review on the topic of somatoform disorders in victims of incest and child abuse, Loewenstein (1990) concludes that the evidence seems compelling that an antecedent history of childhood sexual abuse should be studied as one of the important environmental factors related to the development of somatization disorder. In an interesting article published in the *Journal of the American Medical Association* in 1953, Cohen et al. concluded from a study of women in New England that women diagnosed with hysteria (the diagnosis today would be somatization disorder) had more operations than did the control subjects (3.8 versus 1.9). He comments that no evidence is available to suggest that surgical treatment of hysteria is beneficial.

In a study of 151 women attending a pain clinic, Haber and Roos (1985) found that 53% of the women were physically and/or sexually abused. Abdominal (pelvic pain) and headache subjects revealed the largest percentage of abused women. They comment:

> Psychologically, the abused women used somatization and denial as their primary coping style compared to the nonabused group. Even though abused women had vegetative signs of depression, their denial of psychologic problems was highly significant compared to the nonabused group. (p. 892)

In a study of 135 chronic pain patients, Wurtele, Kaplan, and Keairnes (1990) found that 39% of the women and 7% of the men reported childhood sexual abuse. They comment that more research on the connection between chronic pain and sexual abuse is needed to further elucidate how an experience of childhood abuse might lead to pain complaints in adulthood.

In a recent review article, Laws (1993) noted that available literature on a history of sexual abuse and its role in women's medical problems is sparse. She noted that many studies lack methodological rigor, but that data suggest that a history of sexual abuse in childhood is common in women with a history of chronic pain (especially pelvic pain), functional bowel disorders, eating disorders, obesity, and alcohol abuse. In addressing the utilization of medical care by abused women, Bergman, Brismar, and Nordin (1992) note that traumatic injuries may not be the only consequence of violence. They found that abused women had more hospital admissions than controls in all age groups.

In a study of 523 women attending a primary care health center, 26% indicated a history of sexual abuse before the age of 16. These abused women reported significantly more venereal disease, treatment of pelvic inflammatory disease, and surgical evaluation of pelvic pain than the nonabused group of women (Lechner et al., 1993). The sexual abuse victims indicated more problems in respiratory, gastrointestinal, musculoskeletal, neurological, and gynecologic categories than did the nonabused women.

In my study, I found that women identifying sexual and/or physical abuse were diagnosed with more chronic illness than women denying abuse (67%, compared with 25%) (Radomsky, 1992). In addition, the women identifying abuse also reported more lifetime surgeries (3.3, compared with 1.75).

Even with these reports, which certainly don't represent extensive research, it seems logical to pursue the relationship between chronic pain-medical problems and abuse. In addition, given the total picture of abuse and the relationship to psychiatric problems and injury, it would seem reasonable for physicians to pursue a history of abuse. In a recent study on victimization experiences, it was found that most patients favor inquiry about abuse and believe physicians can help with these problems. Physicians believed they could help although they frequently did not inquire. In the study only 7% of the patients had ever been asked about physical abuse and only 6% had been asked about sexual abuse (Friedman et al, 1992). Likewise in a study of domestic violence in a community practice it was found that of 394 women in the study, the lifetime rate of physical abuse was 38.8%. Only six women in the sample had ever been asked about abuse by their physicians (Hamberger, Saunders, and Hovey, 1992). Sugg and Inui (1992), in a survey of primary care physicians' attitudes about domestic violence, found physicians exploring violence in the clinical setting analogous to opening Pandora's box. The physicians experienced lack of comfort, fear of offending, powerlessness, and problems because of time constraints. In a qualitative study aimed at identifying problems and potential solutions encountered by family physicians in the identification and treatment of wife abuse, Brown, Lent, and Sas (1993) found that a catch phrase for all focus groups regarding the treatment of wife abuse was, "You don't identify what you can't treat." In a retrospective study of female trauma patients presenting in an emergency department, it was found that introducing a protocol designed to detect injuries caused by battering increased the identification of battered women from 5.6% to 30% of trauma patients. However, in an eight-year follow-up it was found that the identification of battered women had reverted to the preprotocol level (McLeer et al. 1989). They comment that education is not enough.

But professionals are increasingly recognizing that a history of sexual or physical abuse is a part of the story for many women with difficult health problems. In a recent editorial in the *Journal of the American Medical Association*, Flitcraft notes:

> The report from the American Medical Association (AMA) Council on Scientific Affairs reviews the epidemiology and clinical dimensions of rape, physical and sexual assaults in marital, cohabiting, and dating relationships, and the longterm effects of child sexual abuse–unveiling women's vulnerability to violence across the life span. The common denominator for women of all ages is that social partners–not strangers–pose the greatest threat of violence. In other words, the predominance of assaults on women occurs within ongoing familial, social, and domestic relationships. As a result, female victims of abuse present a distinct "adult trauma history" typified by recurrent injuries generally accompanied by sexual assault, threats, and verbal abuse. . . . As the medical profession participates in violence prevention and intervention efforts, advances in knowledge, skills, and attitudes are bound to follow. This change will prompt a deeper understanding of the abuse of control and authority in our own professional–and personal–lives. (1992, pp. 3194-95)

What does all of this mean for women–the abuse health issue and physician behavior? There are several ways to look at the above information. We are just beginning to see the relationship of abuse to actual injury, and physical injury–broken bones, lacerations, and wounds–are problems physicians readily recognize to be their concern. And yet doctors have been profoundly slow to respond to these injuries with any recognition of the story behind the injury. The relationship of abuse to psychological problems is now readily recognized, although historically, dating back to Freud, this was not the case. But the business of chronic pain problems and vague health issues and the relationship to abuse is more oblique, more difficult for patient and physician to see or understand. Certainly the research evidence is sparse and we don't really know what this connection between chronic pain and abuse is all about. Furthermore, we don't know whether identifying a history of victimization "helps or hurts" the person and whether the outcome for the chronic pain problem is improved. Because we don't have the research data yet, the cautious physician can proceed as usual, and wait for further evidence. And wait for further research on the right way to detect and intervene when a history of sexual or physical abuse is part of the women's chronic pain story.

WOMEN, RESEARCH, AND ABUSE

But in the meantime women in pain might seriously question whether they can wait. They need to question how long it will be before the right research is done. Unfortunately, even for those health problems women experience that fit nicely into the biomedical model, the research data has been lacking. Only recently has attention been given to the way in which women have been regularly excluded from major research projects (Johnson, 1993) and the way women and men are treated differently even when similar diseases exist. For example, men are more likely to be given dialysis than women and men are more likely to receive a kidney transplant in every age category (Kjellstrand and Logan, 1987). In the group between ages 46 and 60, women have only half the chance of receiving a transplant as men the same age (Kjellstrand, 1988). Doctors are 1.6 times more likely to order cytologic tests for lung cancer on men than on women, even though lung cancer is the leading cause of cancer death in women (Wells and Feinstein, 1988). Cardiovascular disease is the number-one killer of women, yet major research studies excluded women. Recent articles have addressed the gender bias in the management of patients with coronary artery disease. The consensus is that men have cardiac catheterizations ordered at a rate higher than women. However, in an editorial, Laskey (1992) questions the differences and asks: bias or good clinical judgment? In a recent Canadian study, Naylor and Levinton (1993) found that women had more serious symptoms before referral but were turned down for coronary revascularization more often than men.

Alternatively, women live longer than men. Why are women so sure they're neglected or receive inappropriate health care? Furthermore, women receive more health care services in general. For example, women undergo more examination, laboratory tests, and blood pressure checks and receive more drug prescriptions and return appointments than men (Verbrugge and Steiner, 1981). This seems confusing. Too few tests on one hand and more tests and drugs on the other hand.

So, what does this mean for women who experience chronic pain with no readily identified organic problem? Realistically, it means no quick answers. Johnson (1993) notes in her position paper on a women's health research agenda that the year 1990 marked the beginning of a decade in which women's health concerns have received unprecedented attention in academic and public policy circles as well as in the media. She further comments that the Society for the Advancement of Women's Health Research regards the recent attention given to women's health research with cautious optimism. She further notes, however, that the Society has heard concerns regarding the reluctance of the research community to embrace psychosocial and behavioral issues as legitimate and important areas of medical and health research. As a result, issues such as substance abuse, sexual assault, domestic violence, eating disorders, low self-esteem, and depression receive inadequate research attention.

Again–what does this mean for women who experience chronic pain problems associated with no identifiable organic cause? It means their problems will have low priority–for research dollars. But it is much more than that.

In a recent article on domestic violence, Warshaw discusses the constraints of the medical model. She comments:

> Observing how women who seek help for abuse-related symptoms are treated in medical settings reveals the limits of the medical model for providing appropriate care. By examining the ways in which medicine is both taught and practiced, we can see how the objectification process intrinsic to its discourse transforms people–in this case women with lives and agency of their own–into patients who fit medical or psychiatric diagnostic categories. By showing how this model functions through techniques that institutionalize socially sanctioned hierarchies of domination and control, techniques

> that mimic the dynamics of abuse and battering, we begin to see why clinicians trained within that framework find it difficult to provide empowering response that would be most supportive to abused women. . . . Ultimately, however, the objectification inherent in the current structure of medicine, continuously reinforced by external factors and internal needs, is played out in the doctor-patient dynamic in ways that subtly diminish the patient and are often abusive and disempowering. This practice makes it not only possible but acceptable to relate to another person as a nonperson. (1993, pp. 75, 78)

To begin to really address gender-based trauma as a serious health problem will require willingness to move out of the biomedical model and begin to recognize the ways the biomedical model protects physicians from their own sense of powerlessness and loss of control when they relate to the abused person. What will need to happen in this culture and in the medical world for this shift to occur?

But for women with chronic pain: where do they go; where are they heard? The medical profession talks about the overutilization of medical services and reluctance of women to speak about their trauma. Rarely, however, does the profession acknowledge the degree to which physicians over centuries have been part of the culture that repeatedly devalues women and their experience, a culture that repeatedly sees women as other and unimportant.

Women who experience chronic pain problems might consider listening to other women–to other women who too were abused, who too felt alone and silenced. They might want to find women who have found a way to be heard. They might want to listen to women who have told their stories of abuse and pain and who have found new interpretations. They might ask: How do we story our lives in different ways?

The following stories are just that–stories. Stories about women in pain. The stories begin with a voice from the past. The remainder of the stories build on the theme of finding the lost voice in contemporary society. In these stories women begin to say different words and explore new ways of being in the world. They are stories where women rearrange the furniture and envision different rooms–stories where the voices of women are heard.

REFERENCES

Bergman, B., Brismar, B., and Nordin, C. (1992). Utilisation of medical care by abused women. *BMJ* 305:27-28.

Brown, J.B., Lent, B., and Sas, G. (1993). Identifying and treating wife abuse. *J Fam Pract* 36:185-191.

Cohen, M.E., Robins, E., Purtell, J., Altmann, M.W., and Reid, D.E. (1953). Excessive surgery in hysteria. *JAMA* 151:977-986.

Domino, J.V. and Haber, J.D. (1987). Prior physical and sexual abuse in women with chronic headache: clinical correlates. *Headache* 27:310-314.

Drossman, D.A., Leserman, J., Nachman, G., Zhiming, L., Gluck, H., Toomey, T.C., and Mitchell, M. (1990). Sexual and physical abuse in women with functional or organic gastrointestinal disorders. *Ann Intern Med* 113:828-833.

Flitcraft, A.H. (1992). Violence, values and gender. *JAMA* 267:3194-3195.

Friedman, L.S., Samet, J.H., Roberts, M.S., Hidlin, M., and Hans, P. (1992). Inquiry about victimization experiences. *Arch Intern Med* 152:1186-1190.

Haber, J.D. and Roos, C. (1985). Effects of spouse abuse and/or sexual abuse in the development and maintenance of chronic pain in women. *Advances in Pain Research and Therapy* 9:889-895.

Hamberger, L.K., Saunders, D.G., and Hovey, M. (1992). Prevalence of domestic violence in community practice and rate of physician inquiry. *Fam Med* 24:283-287.

Harrop-Griffiths, J., Katon, W., Walker, E., Holm, L., Russco, J., and Hickok, L. (1988). The association between chronic pelvic pain, psychiatric diagnoses, and childhood sexual abuse. *Obstet Gynecol* 71:589-594.

Johnson, T.L. (1993). A women's health research agenda. *J Women's Health* 2:95-97.

Kjellstrand, C.M. (1988). Age, sex, and race inequality in renal transplantation. *Arch Intern Med* 148:1305-1309.

Kjellstrand, C.M. and Logan, G.M. (1987). Racial, sexual and age inequalities in chronic dialysis. *Nephron* 45:257-263.

Laskey, W.K. (1992). Gender differences in the management of coronary artery disease: bias or good clinical judgment. *Ann Intern Med* 116:869-871.

Laws, A. (1993). Does a history of sexual abuse in childhood play a role in women's medical problems? A review. *J Women's Health* 2:165-172.

Lechner, M.E., Vogel, M.E., Garcia-Shelton, L.M, Leichter, J.L., and Steibel, K.R. (1993). Self-reported medical problems of adult female survivors of childhood sexual abuse. *J Fam Pract* 36:633-638.

Loewenstein, R.J. (1990). Somatoform disorders in victims of incest and child abuse. In R.P. Kluft (Ed.), *Incest-related syndromes of adult psychopathology* (pp.75-107). Washington: American Psychiatric Press.

McLeer, S.V., Anwar, R.A.H., Herman, S., and Maquiling, K. (1989). Education is not enough: a systems failure in protecting battered women. *Ann Emerg Med* 18:651-653.

Morrison, J. (1989). Childhood sexual histories of women with somatization disorder. *Am J Psychiatry* 146:239-241.

Naylor, C.D. and Levinton, C.M. (1993). Sex-related differences in coronary revascularization practices: the perspective from a Canadian queue management project. *Can Med Assoc J* 149:965-973.

Radomsky, N.A. (1992). The association of parental alcoholism and rigidity with chronic illness and abuse among women. *J Fam Pract* 35:54-60.

Rapkin, A.J., Kames, L.D., Darke, L.L., Stampler, F.M., and Naliboff, B.D. (1990). History of physical and sexual abuse in women with chronic pelvic pain. *Obstet Gynecol* 76:92-96.

Reiter, R.C., Shakerin, L.R., Gambone, J.C., and Milburn, A.K. (1991). Correlation between sexual abuse and somatization in women with somatic and non-somatic chronic pelvic pain. *Am J Obstet Gynecol* 165:104-109.

Sugg, N.K. and Inui, T. (1992). Primary care physicians' response to domestic violence: opening Pandora's box. *JAMA* 267:3157-3160.

Toomey, T.C., Hernandez, J.T., Gittelman, D.F., and Hulka, J.F. (1993). Relationship of sexual and physical abuse to pain and psychological assessment variables in chronic pelvic pain patients. *Pain* 53:105-109.

Verbrugge, L.M. and Steiner, R.P. (1981). Physician treatment of men and women patients: sex bias or appropriate care? *Med Care* 19:609-632.

Walker, E.A., Katon, W.J., Roy-Byrne, P.P., Jemelka, R.P., and Russo, J. (1993). Histories of sexual victimization in patients with irritable bowel syndrome or inflammatory bowel disease. *Am J. Psychiatry* 150: 1502-1506.

Warshaw, C. (1993). Domestic violence: challenges to medical practice. *J Women's Health* 2:73-80.

Wells, C.K. and Feinstein, A.R. (1988). Detection bias in the diagnostic pursuit of lung cancer. *Am J Epidemiol* 128:869-871.

Wurtele, S.K., Kaplan, G.M., and Keairnes, M. (1990). Childhood sexual abuse among chronic pain patients. *Clin J Pain* 6:110-113.

PART II.
LOST VOICES:
WOMEN IN THE DOCTOR'S OFFICE

I felt as if there was a loud noise of something shattering on the hard floor, there between me and Adam and our baby and the doctor. But there was only a ringing of silence. Which seemed oddly, after a moment, like the screaming of monkeys.

–Alice Walker, *Possessing the Secret of Joy*

Chapter 8

Anna O: A Voice from Medical "Herstory"

> . . . When we consider the intimate connection of the uterus with the great sympathetic nervous system, and the frequent deleterious impression of the stomach, heart and head reflexly therefrom by the way of this nervous connection, it is but carrying the same reflex process but one step farther when we assert its reflex influence over the organs of the voice. If good singers have themselves noticed this, at their regular monthly periods, and so have abstained as much as possible from the critical exercise of their voices at these regularly recurring periods, and many have so told me that they have noticed the prejudicial influence of these periods over their voices, then it stands to reason that an inflamed or congested uterus will, at other times, also prejudiciously affect the organs of voice and song.
>
> –*The Journal of the American Medical Association* (July 9, 1892)

THE STORY OF BERTHA PAPPENHEIM

This is the story of Anna O, Paul Berthold, and Bertha Pappenheim. Anna O–the lost voice, the name given to her by her doctor. Paul Berthold–the false voice, the pseudonym she used. Bertha Pappenheim–the empowered voice that she found.

The story begins with Anna O. The setting is the late nineteenth century in Paris. The place is a hospital complex for the mentally disturbed. The topic of study is hysteria. But first, a bit of history about hysteria, that disease once thought to arise in the womb.

Hysteria affected upper- and upper-middle-class women almost exclusively and had been around for centuries. The problem occurred in North America and Europe. Hysteria took on many variations: hysterical coughing, screaming, fits and fainting, loss of appetite, crying, etc. Doctors could find no organic basis for the problem.

For various reasons, the famous French neurologist, Jean-Martin Charcot, decided to study hysteria and in so doing gave credibility to serious investigation of a problem that had generally been relegated to the popular healers. Charcot's approach emphasized careful observation and classification. His lectures and demonstrations attracted many important people of the day. These included the famous doctors: Pierre Janet, William James, and Sigmund Freud. The men of science listened to the women and likely achieved collaboration with their patients to an extent not previously known in the medical world.

Anna O was the name given to Bertha Pappenheim by her doctor. She was one of the more celebrated "cases" of hysteria. Little is known about her early childhood, except that she was passionately fond of her father. Doctors described her as having a "double personality" and as having a "magnetic illness." Her doctor was Joseph Breuer who collaborated with Freud.

For several years, Dr. Breuer regularly saw Anna O. Anna described events with Dr. Breuer as the "talking cure." However, after two years of therapy, Dr. Breuer abruptly ended his treatment with Anna. Anna O worsened and the crisis resulted in her hospitalization, where she remained ill for several more years. To glimpse the complexity of events surrounding the termination of her therapy, a quick walk through medical history is required.

Medicine as a profession requiring university training began in the Middle Ages. Because universities were closed to women this meant doctors were men.

Women as healers, however, existed long before the Middle Ages (Salk et al., 1992). The healing arts were almost exclusively in the hands of women–the priestesses–in Assyria, Egypt, Greece, and Sumer until the third millennium (2000-3000 B.C.). Midwifery was quite advanced by 1550 B.C. in Egypt. But civilizations come and go.

The conversion of the Roman Empire to Christianity changed attitudes towards woman as healers. By the fourteenth century the Church decreed that any woman who healed others without having studied was duly a witch and should suffer death. And so, the witch trials. The Church, law, and medicine came together in the fifteenth and sixteenth centuries and executed thousands of "witches." Women made up 85% of those executed and were mainly peasant women and female healers.

Female healers in North America were not eliminated with the same degree of violence. However, the American medical profession outlawed midwifery in the late nineteenth century, and "His-medicine" was established. Women's role became that of customer or employee of the doctor.

Back to Anna O.

As the study of hysteria progressed, the possibility that sexual trauma played a role in the disease became a line of inquiry persued by Freud and his followers. By 1896 Freud believed he had found the source of the problem and published a report on 18 case studies entitled "The Aetiology of Hysteria." However, if he really believed his patients, then the extent of childhood sexual abuse would have seemed overwhelming. The political climate of the day dictated an inability to accept this information. Freud later retracted the "seduction theory." He concluded that many of the stories were women's fantasies and not their reality (Loewenstein, 1990). He developed other theories.

It's not difficult to imagine Dr. Breuer's dilemma: the dilemma of a man who wanted the prestige of his profession; the dilemma of a man who wanted to help his patient but who likely experienced confusion with regard to Anna O. At any rate, Dr. Breuer for whatever reason, abruptly stopped Anna's therapy. At the same time, the learned men of the day were unable to acknowledge the reality of the abuse in women's lives. Of course it didn't help Anna O. It's difficult to imagine how she eventually found her voice. But she did. Eventually she left the hospital. Eventually, against all obstacles, she translated into German an important piece of information about women. She translated Mary Wollstonecraft's work entitled "A Vindication of the Rights of Women." She used her pseudonym–Paul Berthold–for this project. She also wrote a play, *Women's Rights* (Herman, 1992).

Sometimes we think the women's movement started in the '60s. We forget the courageous women in the late 1800s and early 1900s who struggled desperately for a life of meaning and activity. We've never even heard about the long lost past where women were the healers. We forget our recent history, with the extremes in the social system that existed during the time of Anna O–the chronic sickness of the upper-middle-class lady of leisure contrasted with the working-lower-class women of the day who received inadequate nutrition and rest and suffered from contagious diseases and complications of childbirth. Tuberculosis was more common in women than in men, a fact sometimes viewed as proof of women's defective physiology.

But back to Anna O, or Paul Berthold. She eventually surfaced as Bertha Pappenheim–her real name. She managed to climb out of the big pool of social injustice and she became a prominent organizer for women. She campaigned against the sexual exploitation of women and children. People remembered her passion and spirit.

Incredibly–against insurmountable odds–Bertha found her voice.

I'd like to dismiss this story. This was 100 years ago. Doctors are very sophisticated in diagnosis and treatment now in comparison to the past. But–some questions to think about. In what way does the medical profession continue to determine which problems are important enough to study? Is the medical profession any more prepared to listen to stories of abuse, particularly against women, today than they were in 1890? What part of Bertha's story do you identify with?

REFERENCES

Herman, J.L. (1992). A Forgotten History. In J.L. Herman (Ed.), *Trauma and Recovery* (pp. 7-32). USA:Basic Books.

Loewenstein, R.J. (1990). Somatoform Disorders in Victims of Incest and Child Abuse. In R.P. Kluft (Ed.), *Incest-Related Syndromes of Adult Psychopathology* (pp. 75 -111). Washington, DC: American Psychiatric Press.

Salk, H., Sanford, W., Swenson, N., and Luce, J.D. (1992). The Politics of Women and Medical Care. In *The New Our Bodies, Ourselves* (pp.6 51-698). New York: Simon and Schuster Inc.

Chapter 9

Jenny: My Baby

> In the old wrecked car, in the smelly old Buick at the back of the lot, Marya knew how to go into stone; how to shut her mind off, to see nothing without closing her eyes.
>
> –Joyce Carol Oates, *Marya*

JENNY'S STORY

Jenny at Age 16

I glanced at the chart before entering the room. A new patient. I noticed the birth date. Young. Some 16-year-old women seem to instantly fill the room–their unusual clothes, exotic hairstyles, and makeup make it impossible to not notice them. Jenny looked down. She seemed invisible. I can't remember any details about her hair or clothes. I recall she seemed thin.

"Hi, I'm Dr. Radomsky," I said, hoping to get some eye contact. She looked up.

"I'd like to go on the pill," she said quickly, looking nervous as she squeezed her hands.

"Okay, let's talk," I said.

I asked the usual questions. It sounded as if she was lucky she wasn't already pregnant. She smoked cigarettes. She lived with her mother, stepfather, and two younger sisters. She seemed healthy. No headaches, no liver problems, no phlebitis, etc. I did the usual tests–pap test, cultures, blood pressure check, etc. I talked about the pill–how to take it, side effects, reinforced the need for condoms–advised her to stop the smoking. I gave her the sample starting pack of birth control pills and suggested she return in a few months for a recheck and prescription for the pill.

Jenny Returns Eight Months Later

Of course I had not realized Jenny failed to return for follow-up. I glanced at the chart as I entered the room eight months later, wondering what she was up to.

"I think I'm pregnant," she quickly blurted out.

I looked at the chart again. "But aren't you taking the pill?"

"When I finished those samples, I just stopped. I broke up with my boyfriend. It seemed pointless to take the pill. Besides I had funny bleeding. I didn't like the pill."

"Okay," I said, "but you think you're pregnant."

"Yes. My period's three weeks late. I feel sick. I've met someone else and I didn't get started on the pills again."

"Let's do a pregnancy test," I suggested, "and then we'll go from there." I filled the requisition and Jenny went to the lab. Jenny returned. Not too surprising. Positive.

"That means you're pregnant," I said to Jenny.

Her head dropped. She rubbed her knees. She squeezed her hands.

I waited.

She looked up. Her expression–calm, intense, resigned, but sad. "I thought so," she said. "I've already thought about it. I know I'm keeping the baby."

I nodded, sensing she anticipated certain questions. "Have you talked to anyone yet?"

"No."

"Okay," I continued, "can you talk to your parents?"

"I can talk to my mother," she said, "but I already know I'll move out. I can live with a friend."

She seemed to have figured a lot out already. I noticed the intensity of her eyes and the look of resignation on her face and realized she seemed older than 16. But I suspected she would struggle with the pregnancy just as other 16-year-old women did. This time I made sure she understood what I meant about return appointments and her responsibilities in this pregnancy. As we talked I realized that she desperately wanted this pregnancy.

Her pregnancy didn't go well. Bleeding started around eight weeks. The ultrasound showed a viable pregnancy, but the scan suggested problems, though it was too early to clearly determine the situation. She lost weight. She worried. She moved in with a friend and contacted the social worker. The bleeding settled. The scan at 12 weeks looked optimistic. The fetus had grown, although there still seemed to be a problem, likely with the placenta. At 17 weeks she could feel her uterus through the abdominal wall. Sometimes she even smiled. And then the bleeding started again. The scan showed more problems with the placenta. I tried to explain to her that we couldn't predict the outcome. This clearly was a case of "wait and see."

She made it to 20 weeks. One morning the cramping started in earnest. I got the call from the case room.

I arrived. Jenny looked frightened.

I checked her. She was almost fully dilated.

"Jenny," I said, "you're losing this pregnancy. Your baby is too little–there is no hope at this point."

She nodded and grasped the sheets as another contraction gripped her.

It was over with quickly. The fetus–perfectly formed–was dead. The placenta didn't look normal.

Jenny sobbed.

The next morning I found Jenny in her bed with covers pulled to her shoulders. Her sad brown eyes stared nowhere.

"It's not fair," she said. "I really wanted that baby."

"I know. It's going to hurt. You've lost something important."

Tears filled her eyes.

"Please let me out of here. I can't stand this place–all these mothers and babies."

I checked her. "You can leave today, Jenny, but see me in the office this week." She looked relieved.

Jenny came to the office, went back on birth control pills, talked about catching up in school, and then–I didn't realize it–she moved. Relatives in Kamloops came to her rescue.

I wondered. Did I fail to explain the birth control pill properly? But I've seen so many young women in this situation–obviously the issue is more complex than that. I feel frustrated. I thought young women were supposed to have some advantages. I feel annoyed. Jenny seems irresponsible. I want to tell her about our grandmothers and great-grandmothers. They had their own unreliable methods of birth control–cocoa butter, strange douches. Can't Jenny see anything? And I feel guilty. Likely I have no idea what this is all about for Jenny. How can I be so judgmental? I feel confused. I want to talk to someone, anyone, about these young women. But so often the view is just that they're failures. And then when Jenny lost the pregnancy–I could see her pain and anguish. It bothered me that I felt so distant–so not wanting to understand her dilemma. I want Jenny and her problems to go away. I just want young women who are organized and getting on with their life to see me. I don't want to ask difficult questions.

Jenny at Age 19

Jenny returned from Kamloops. I glanced at the chart as I opened the door of the examining room. Jenny looked thinner, older, and more intense than I remembered her to be. She quickly filled me in.

"I moved. I lived with my aunt for a year and then worked in Kamloops. I decided to go back to school. That's why I'm back in Red Deer. Anyway, you don't want to hear all of that," she quickly continued. "I've been having a lot of problems this last year–the doctors can't figure it out."

"So, what's been happening," I said.

"It started a year ago. First, I got–you know–that disease chlamy," she hesitated. "Chlamydia," I said.

"Yes, that's it. Anyway, I got antibiotics three times. But I keep having pain–you know down here," and she pointed to her lower pelvic area. "And sex hurts. Actually, I don't have a boyfriend right now," she continued, "and don't worry, I'm on the pill." She talked faster than usual. "But it's the pain. I'm sure there's something wrong. I even had one of those operations–you know where they make that little cut below your belly-button."

"Um–you had a laparoscopy," I suggested.

"That's it. And they said everything looked okay."

"Sounds like the last year hasn't been much fun," I said. "Are you having pain right now?"

"Not really," she said. "It comes and goes."

"Okay," I continued, "let's do it this way. I think we need to spend more time talking before we just plunge into more tests. Since you're not hurting now," and she nodded, "could you book for a longer appointment next week and we'll try to sort things out a bit more." She agreed. "And of course if the pain suddenly escalates, come back sooner," I advised.

She returned. We first talked about the pain. There was no definite pattern but the pain occurred to some degree every week. Every day she thought about the pain.

I told her I wanted to carefully go over her family history and past history, even though I realized she thought I probably knew everything already.

"Your parents–still healthy?" She nodded. And then I realized it was a stepfather and mother.

"Just a minute," I said. "Do you know anything about your natural father?"

"No–Mom never talked about him. He left before I was born."

"Oh–and then your mother remarried and had your two sisters?"

"Uh, uh."

"So how old were you when your mother married?"

"Oh, I was eight. She was so happy when she got married. And then, she had my sisters right away. I never really felt like part of that family."

We continued and reviewed more family medical history. I realized I had never asked about abuse or alcoholism.

"I ask everyone these questions," I commented as I continued.

"Have you ever in the past or now been concerned about your parents use of alcohol or drugs?"

She looked puzzled. "Well–my stepfather drinks a lot–I don't know. Seems like he's drinking more than he used too. I know Mom hates his drinking."

"Um," I murmured as I decided not to pursue the topic more at the moment. "And Jenny were you ever aware of any sexual or physical abuse to yourself or anyone else in the family?"

Her eyes dropped instantly. She looked uncomfortable.

I waited.

She looked up and nodded.

"Have you ever talked to anyone about this?"

She shook her head.

"Do you want to talk about it now?"

"It was my stepfather," she replied. "But it was mostly when I was 10–maybe 12–he had his hands all over me any chance he could get. Then it stopped. He just kept looking at me." She seemed to be thinking. "Remember when I got pregnant? I was so glad to get out of that house. I couldn't live there anymore. I can't stand the man."

"Um–yes, I remember," I said.

"Anyway, I don't think about it. It's gone–done–over."

I continued. "I always ask this, Jenny, because I think sometimes these experiences affect us in ways we don't really understand. Sometimes it helps to talk about it. You can come back anytime and we could talk more if you wanted to."

She nodded. "It's over."

I finished the history and then did a physical check, including repeating the cultures. "I'm not sure what I'll find, Jenny," I said. "Could you come back in a week and we'll go over the results?" I advised her that her exam seemed completely normal. "Well, there's something wrong. I'll be back," she said.

When she returned a week later she looked less anxious.

"So, how's school?" I asked.

"School is going amazingly well. This course takes me one year and with any luck I'll have a better job."

"How's the pain?"

"It's there."

I reviewed her results. "Your cultures are completely okay. You have no evidence of infection."

"So, what's wrong?"

"I'm not sure," I said, "but I've excluded major concerns with these cultures and because the laparoscopy was normal I'm reluctant to pursue more investigation. I've been wondering though," I continued, "how much do you think about that chlamydia infection?"

"The chlamydia–for sure, I think about it. All the magazines have something in them about chlamydia and wrecking your tubes. I keep thinking that I'll never get pregnant again. I'm scared. You know I really want a baby someday."

"Um."

Our eyes met. "Maybe this all fits together, somehow," I suggested. "I know you want a baby sometime. It's true that chlamydia can cause problems with the tubes, but in many cases there is no damage. There is an incredible amount of chlamydia out there and of course I see women all the time getting pregnant when they've had a history of chlamydia."

"Really?"

"Yes, but it makes sense that you're worried. And until you actually have a healthy baby I think you'll likely have some anxiety about all of this."

"Um, so what about the pain?"

"I don't know. I would suggest we go slow. You've had the major tests. We can reassess the problem if the pain changes."

"You think my pain isn't real?"

"Not at all," I said. "I just think there aren't easy answers to everything. You've packed a lot into your life already."

She nodded.

"Could you come back in a month and we could reassess this?" She looked somewhat unsure but agreed.

"Are you comfortable with this approach?"

"I think so," she said.

Nine months later she returned. "I think I'm pregnant," she said. "I did one of those home pregnancy things. But, it's okay. I want to be pregnant. And this boyfriend is different. He treats me okay."

She went to the lab for the pregnancy test. Positive. "You're pregnant," I said. She put her hands over her face and then suddenly looked up at me. "I'm so happy. I want this baby so bad." I had never seen Jenny look quite like that before. Relief and joy in one package.

This time the pregnancy went well. When the boyfriend moved out after two months, Jenny wasn't terribly upset. At this point she had finished school. She had just started a job. This path she had clearly chosen.

I wondered. When Jenny returned from Kamloops and told the story about pelvic pain, I knew I had to approach this pain problem from many different perspectives. I'm acutely aware of the many organic problems that can produce pelvic pain–endometriosis, infections, ovarian cysts, etc. However, I wanted desperately to convey to Jenny that I could not approach her chronic pain problem with black-and-white thinking. But how could I convey to Jenny that I really heard her? I know she feels her pain. I feel so frustrated sometimes in my own struggle to move away from either/or thinking. I'm already focused on her lost pregnancy. Has she resolved this pain? I feel my own sense of helplessness with Jenny. Did I support her appropriately when she lost that pregnancy? I simply want to fix her. I wish this pelvic pain problem had an easy label.

When I asked Jenny about the abuse I got information but she seemed to close the door to more dialogue. That's frustrating, but I know I must respect Jenny's space. Likewise, I'm sure that even though this question shifted the thinking further than she could handle at that moment I still hoped something registered with her. But I don't know. I know that pelvic pain can be associated with abuse issues. If I find ways to understand how abuse affects us and find ways to encourage healing from abuse, will there be less pelvic pain? I don't know. Those research studies haven't been done.

When I asked about chlamydia and whether she thought about it, I sensed a new direction in our conversation. I'm sure sometimes that questions with my patients really do open doors for new ways to think together. I just wish I understood this process better.

Intuitively, I know that Jenny is not terribly connected with other humans. After all, we learn about relationships first in our families and I'm sure Jenny learned more about disconnecting that connection while growing up. I sensed she never felt like she was part of the family. I wondered. What about Jenny's need for the baby? I sensed she needed to create her own baby to ensure some connection. That idea seems too simple. But is it?

Jenny Has a Baby

This time Jenny's pregnancy went well. She stopped smoking. She took care of herself. The pelvic pain problem seemed to disappear! She had the usual aches and pains of pregnancy but managed to cope well. And then–the day arrived.

"Here comes another one," Jenny said carefully as she breathed in deeply.

"Okay, let it build," Amy, her nurse, coached her. "Three good pushes this time." Jenny nodded.

I noticed the beads of sweat on Jenny's forehead. Repeatedly, she pushed her dark long curls off her forehead. Her lips were dry. Her makeup had long disappeared. Her eyes, brown and intense, focused on Amy's face and then she pushed.

"Wonderful, Jenny," I said. "I can see the baby's hair." The black hair peeked from the vagina. The opening expanded. More hair pressed forward. Jenny pushed again. The baby's head pressed tightly onto the opening. The skin stretched paper thin, tense against the black hair.

"Take another breath, Jenny, and give one more push," I encouraged her.

And then she cried out, "I can't. Damn, this hurts." She moaned–almost yelled–and seemed to pull her body away from the intensity and pressure.

"Slow your breathing," Amy said.

I noticed that Jenny continued to squeeze Amy's hand. Amy's hand disappeared in Jenny's grasp and I wondered–how much pressure can a hand take before it becomes mush.

Jenny breathed deeply. "Ice. I need ice," she said.

Amy reached for the pitcher. Usually husbands or boyfriends or sometimes mothers or friends play that role. Jenny's boyfriend left shortly after she became pregnant. Jenny closed her eyes, as she munched on the ice. A minute passed. She looked more relaxed. Sometimes three minutes between contractions seems like forever. Sometimes it doesn't seem long enough.

I moved from the end of the bed to Jenny's side. "Jenny, can you open your eyes," I said. She nodded, and when her eyes focused on mine I continued. "You're so close, Jenny. Next time, when you feel that burning pain and sense you'll explode and tear, think about making the pressure just a bit bigger. You can do it."

She nodded and closed her eyes.

"Okay, I feel it coming again. Help me," she said.

With the first push the vagina quickly opened as the mass of hair stretched the opening.

"Great, Jenny," I said as she continued to push.

She took another breath. Her face looked flushed. Everything about her seemed focused. She quickly pushed again. This time the baby's head had not disappeared. The pressure persisted and the head pressed forward until she began to tear.

"Just pant," I said.

And then the baby's head came out. I quickly checked for a cord around the neck.

"I need to push again," Jenny said.

"Go ahead, you'll feel some pressure with the shoulders."

"You have a girl, Jenny," I said, as I placed the baby on her abdomen.

"A girl. I have a girl. I can't believe it." she said. She touched her baby's face. "Is she okay?" she quickly asked.

The baby cried out while Amy rubbed and dried her.

"She looks fine," I said, as I clamped and cut the cord.

"I just can't believe it," she said again, as she dropped her head back onto the bed, completely exhausted.

Silence fell over all of us. Another life–another miracle.

Amy placed the baby under the heat lamp and continued to dry her. The baby's noises reassured all of us. Wonderful sounds.

"What's happening?" Jenny questioned with fear in her voice.

I noticed the gushes of blood. I quickly felt for her uterus through the abdominal wall. I could feel it harden. "It's just your placenta," I said reassuring her. "You'll feel some pressure and cramping until you've passed it."

"That hurts," she said as she pushed on my hand against her abdomen. "I thought I was done."

"That's it," I said, as the placenta came out.

"I'm so tired," she said.

"You did a great job, Jenny. Congratulations."

"What a lovely baby," Amy exclaimed. Jenny looked over at Amy. They both smiled. I sensed they shared a special moment.

Jenny closed her eyes. I quickly repaired the tear. Amy organized Jenny's bed while I checked the baby.

"Is she okay?" Jenny questioned again.

Her little hands and feet were wrinkled. Her skin seemed blotchy and red. Her pointed head told a story of a tight squeeze. But it all added up to perfection.

I went to Jenny's side. I touched her hand.

"Congratulations, Jenny. She's perfect."

Amy wrapped the baby and placed her in Jenny's arms. Jenny stroked her face. "My baby. A girl. I can't believe it."

Amy organized Jenny for nursing the baby. I wrote notes and then told Jenny I would see her in the morning.

I glanced at my watch as I walked down the hall–5:00 a.m. I seemed wide awake. I wondered about Jenny. I couldn't keep other pictures from my mind. I remembered five years ago when Jenny was 16 and lost the pregnancy. The last few years had been so traumatic for Jenny. What a relief to have everything go well.

I wondered. I had a strong sense of Jenny's strength throughout the birth process. Young women regularly seem to be choosing pregnancy when they've come from families where family relationships have been difficult. What does this mean? Certainly Jenny had more control over the connection with her daughter than in past family relationships. How important is that to Jenny? But certainly she must have felt very alone giving birth–yet she wanted the pregnancy. She worried about her fertility. I wondered. What about pelvic pain and fertility or lack of fertility? What about pelvic pain and fear? Do women talk about these fears to each other, to their doctors, to anyone? Or how silenced do women feel?

Two Years After the Birth

Jenny arrived one day without Tammy, her daughter. She had coped well, but it had not been easy. Her job barely supported them. But she managed. The pelvic pain issue occasionally surfaced but never developed into a greater problem. She looked particularly upset that day.

"I need help," she said.

"Tammy is driving me crazy. I'm scared. Sometimes I'm sure I'm going to hit her. I don't want anything to happen to her. I worry all the time. Someone will hurt her. I'm afraid it might be me."

We talked.

"You're a brave woman, Jenny," I said. "I can see you want

something for Tammy that is different from what you had growing up."

She agreed.

I became somewhat philosophical.

"It's interesting how it works. If we want something different for our kids than what we had, generally it means we have to look back first. You grew up with someone always squashing you–abuse in many different ways. Your tendency is going to be to squash Tammy as well, or to just let her have her own way with everything."

"I know," she said quickly, "that's why I'm here."

We talked about various therapists who could help her.

She sighed. "I wish there was an easier way but I guess there isn't. Okay, I'll call that therapist."

"Good," I commented, and then realized I was thinking out loud. "Sometimes I would like a magic pill, too. But there isn't one. I know you'll find answers in therapy. You're motivated."

Jenny left–determined to find another way. There would be many more chapters in Jenny's story. That day, she started a new one.

I felt completely focused on Jenny in that visit. I was so aware of her struggle to find answers. I could see that Jenny was trying to break the cycle of abuse. I wondered if she talked to me that day because I had raised the abuse issue three years ago? I didn't know. I realized Jenny had taught me so much. I wanted to talk out loud to her about this but I thought that would be inappropriate. Perhaps at a later point I could share this with her. My job was to support Jenny–to give her space to express her voice. I wondered. As Jenny's voice became stronger what would Jenny continue to tell us?

Chapter 10

Elaine: The Two Picture Books

> First there was Janet, whose bloke had been "In Love" with her, had chased her for months till she'd finally come round, as they say; come to her senses, he'd said. And Paul had been ever so romantic, insisting on a church wedding, white dress, whisking her off to a grand honeymoon. Janet don't talk about Love no more though–bit difficult when half your teeth been knocked out, and all the other bits of your body knocked in.
>
> –Ravinder Randhawa, *War of the Worlds*

ELAINE JOHNSEN'S STORY

Elaine chatted and filled me in on the news since her last visit. She needed more birth control pills, needed her pap test repeated, and just wanted to make sure everything was okay. I hadn't seen Elaine for several years. She had been busy, taking classes and taking care of her two boys. Her body was fine. The news centered on her family.

"The divorce should come through next month," she said.

"So how have things been," I said, remembering that I had seen her just twice since she left Ralph. I vividly recalled her visit when she had been in the shelter. She had bruises on her neck and arms, and the depression and anxiety were overwhelming.

"Not great, but I'll be glad when the divorce is settled."

And then she started to talk quickly. I realized I was seeing a part of Elaine that I had never observed before. The Elaine sitting in front of me had short blond hair, clear blue eyes and a tall body that could be on any magazine cover. As she talked, she gestured, smiled, frowned, and occasionally stopped and looked quiet. That pensive, anxious woman that I had known five years ago was gone.

"What really bugs me is that he's trying to get custody of the boys. I can't believe it. He hardly visits now. He keeps up the payments but that's about it. I know he just wants his mother to have the boys. Next year Paul will be in the first grade and Joey will be in play school. He hardly knows them. And when he does take them for a day, inevitably the kids come back upset and anxious."

"I've heard that before," I said.

"But you know, I'm scared. The last time in court the judge looked asleep. He sat there with his hand on his chin. I don't think he heard a word that was said. And Ralph can be so convincing."

"Ummm."

"Sometimes I feel so frustrated. Ralph comes across as Mr. Nice Guy. He can convince the best of them. That psychologist Ralph saw a few years ago didn't have a clue. I couldn't believe what happened. After Ralph went to the psychologist twice, he refused to go anymore. The psychologist called me and told me he couldn't see what the problem was. He thought Ralph was doing just fine. Meanwhile, Ralph threatened and intimidated like you wouldn't believe. He only got the gun out once, but that was enough. He just had to look across the room at me and I could feel my throat tighten. You know when I used to come in with those chest pains–even ended up in emergency a few times–you kept thinking it had something to do with that heart valve. Well, I think it was just about Ralph and me. Ralph was always on my case."

"Yes, I remember those things," I said, as I had glimpses of the scared Elaine I used to see but recalled that I had no idea of her dilemma during those visits. And I realized I had never asked. I too had occasionally seen her husband and thought, "he's organized and put together okay." Elaine always seemed to be the one that didn't cope, couldn't care for the kids, and was neurotic, or so it seemed.

"Anyway, I'll be glad to have the divorce settled, and if the judge isn't awake on this one I'll just have to keep going back, because I must have custody of the kids. I know between Ralph and his mother they will bring up everything they can to paint a picture of an incompetent mother."

"Well, you've certainly come a long way, Elaine."

"You can say that."

And she seemed lost in thought for a few minutes and rattled on more. I knew she needed to talk with this divorce business coming up and I think I found myself watching her and marveling at the Elaine that I had never observed before. It was almost as if part of her had never been in my office before. It seemed that there were two Elaines: an Elaine that I could picture in a book labeled "before I left him," and another Elaine in a book labeled "after I left him."

"That time he threatened to kill me and I called the police, I was scared. When I got to the shelter I almost felt guilty. Some of the women had situations so much worse than mine. I really don't think he'd ever use the gun. But I've never told you. Sometimes he drinks. Not often. Twice he got drunk and broke dishes in the kitchen. Never touched me but made a hell of a mess. I knew after I went to the shelter that I could never go back. Thank God for the women that work there. I got so much support. It can seem so humiliating."

"You have so much strength now, Elaine. Just look at you. You are really alive."

"I know. I'll never be that old Elaine again. I know I will get the kids. He cannot destroy me."

Elaine continued to chat as I checked her. I gave her the prescription for more birth control pills. She talked about her courses. In another year she would be finished. With her energy I knew she would continue to put pictures in her second album that would be pictures of a strong and alive Elaine.

Later that day I thought about other Elaines that I knew. Sometimes I only knew about their pictures in one of the albums and sometimes I knew about both albums. But it seemed with all Elaines that the stories were variations on the theme: "Is it possible to be alive–to be healthy–and have no fear?"

OTHER VOICES

Elaine Smalsky

She just appears in the second book. On her first visit she told me about her stomachaches–irritable bowel syndrome it seemed. She felt that everything would be fine now.

"He doesn't know where Sam (her seven-year-old son) and I are," she said, "and the police have reassured me that when he gets out of jail they'll let me know."

I don't think I ever saw Elaine Smalsky without sensing her fear. Her stomach aches and pelvic pain were recurring problems. When she moved away after two years it didn't surprise me. I don't know if she will ever stop running. It seems that I know many Elaine Smalskys. They move to a new town after they leave him, so I see their pictures in the second album. Sometimes they have jobs. Sometimes they are on social assistance and have small children. Sometimes they take classes. Generally, they have headaches, bellyaches, and pain somewhere.

Elaine Graholl

Her story continues to haunt me.

I know about parts of Elaine Graholl's first album. I cared for her during her three pregnancies and I really thought things were fine. Her children always looked cared for. And even though she seemed depressed, anxious, and had headaches at times, Elaine appeared to cope with the tasks required of a busy wife and mother. The day she appeared with her earache is a day I won't forget.

She sat with her hand over her ear. Elaine Graholl was a petite woman with brown curly hair and big brown eyes.

"It's my ear," she said. "It really hurts."

"Have you had any other symptoms? A sore throat or runny nose?"

"No, just my ear."

I could see she was in pain and then noticed the tears forming in her big brown eyes. I quickly checked her. One ear was fine. I looked into the other ear and realized that this was no ear infection. The canal was filled with blood.

"Elaine, what's happened?" I asked as I quickly tuned into the problem. "Has anyone hurt you?"

"He hit me," she said as her eyes dropped, "but he didn't mean to. It's never happened before. It hurts so much."

In retrospect, I don't know if I handled this one right. I quickly reassured her that I could help her with the pain problem and because of the extent of the damage I wanted her to see a specialist. I arranged for someone to see her that afternoon. I also talked briefly about her safety. But I realized as I did so that she didn't want to talk about these issues. I suggested she return in two days.

Elaine Graholl never returned. The specialist sent me a letter and told me he saw her a few times and that her eardrum healed nicely. I don't know if she moved, if she went to another doctor, if she and her husband got counseling, if–if–if there are pictures in Elaine's first album that are Elaine alive and well, or if–if–.

Elaine O'Breen

He never touched her–that is, physically hurt her. When she was depressed and spent three months in the hospital in Calgary when she was in her forties she had overheard him tell the psychiatrist: "Yes, she can come home even if she isn't completely well. She is never any good around the place anyway."

When Elaine told me that years after the event she said: "Isn't it funny–I raised five children–we fought a lot early on but then I just stopped trying–I had to keep the kids organized and fed."

Elaine hasn't left him but I'm beginning to see her before and after picture books. Before, the Elaine that always looked sad; the Elaine with pain somewhere; the Elaine in her fifties, dressed with every item pressed, matched, and perfect. Something about her in those days looked dead, looked as if she was stopped in her tracks, looked as if maybe she was in a show and the director had forgotten to tell her that she had a part.

Now that Elaine was 63, she felt she was running out of time. "I'm not going to leave him, I don't think," she said one day, "but that doesn't stop me from going where I'm going."

And so Elaine had stopped making coffee, was taking courses, was talking to other people, was not listening to his complaints anymore. She wasn't even sure yet if he noticed, but she was seeing her path and nothing could stop her. Elaine looks different now. Her clothes still match but sometimes they're wrinkled–wrinkled as if someone moves in them. Her body still hurts, but Elaine O'Breen can talk these days and that seems to be making a difference.

Elaine Haine

I can see Elaine and her husband in both albums. That's unusual. In the first book they're both unhappy and depressed. It's no mystery that he had headaches and she had stomach pains. It's no mystery that they shared similar childhood stories. Both of them experienced abuse and neglect. It's no mystery that he threatened and she withdrew. It's no mystery that the marriage crumbled as the children grew up.

The miracle was the way they both struggled to get into the second book. They went for joint counseling and individual counseling. He stayed in a hotel the night he worried that he may harm her. He talked about his fears. She talked about her fears. They struggled, sometimes grew apart, and now I occasionally will see one of them. He still looks tired, but that edge of anger is softening. His headaches are less of a problem. Her irritable bowel syndrome remains an issue, but no longer dominates her life. She looks clearer, and sometimes when I see their picture in that second book I almost visualize them balanced–both of them alive.

Elaine Peterson

They called from the women's shelter. "Elaine says you're her doctor. We can't control her here. She's incredibly disruptive. What do you suggest?"

I hardly knew Elaine Peterson. She had been in my office once. I knew she had a difficult history–sexual abuse as a child, disastrous relationships, and a completely unsuccessful track record with doctors. (I gathered that the reason she was in the women's shelter on this occasion was another disastrous relationship–bruises over her arms, breasts, and neck.) She had been labeled borderline personality disorder. Besides many contacts with psychiatrists, she had managed an equally exhaustive record with physicians of all specialties. I was amazed at the number of surgeries she described, and with all of her scars concluded that she was accurate enough. And, of course, even from that first visit, I wondered about the extent of drug and alcohol abuse.

There were no beds on the psychiatric unit the day they called from the shelter. I arranged her admission to a medical unit. She insisted that her abdominal pain was overwhelming. She insisted on narcotics. She became disruptive and unmanageable when these requests were not met. The psychiatrist didn't think she met the criteria for committing her to the mental institution. She calmed down long enough to discharge herself. Four days later I heard that she came to emergency with slashed wrists and alcohol intoxication.

Somehow it seemed that as I looked into the first picture book, I saw a picture of Elaine. Elaine's body swirled around at the bottom of a waterfall. Upstream in the picture I could see many rapids and other waterfalls. Certainly Elaine seemed to be drowning. She couldn't swim. It seemed too late for her to learn to swim–rescue attempts weren't working–and yet I found it difficult to accept that there was so little hope.

Elaine Strawhau

I had just a glimpse of her in the second album. She saw me once. She was on her way to a treatment center in British Columbia. She had fallen and had bruises on her back and leg. It was one of those winters with icy sidewalks. The visit was brief. She had to show me her back and legs and of course I saw the scars.

"Oh, he tried to kill me," she said. "He poured gasoline on me–tried to burn me. And that's why I have scars on my back and legs. I almost died."

I sensed she was still running but she hoped things would get better if she went to the treatment center.

Elaine Booth

On a recent visit Elaine shared more of her story with me–all pictures in the first album. Elaine is 54 years old, works as a secretary and tries desperately to support her two sons and one daughter in their quest for higher education. Her husband works out of town and as Elaine says, "fortunately he isn't home much." But his salary is crucial in terms of the children. Elaine's salary barely buys food. I know all of these details about Elaine's life. I also listen regularly to her concerns about her health. On the surface it seems so simple–Elaine is significantly overweight. If Elaine would just address some life-style issues–exercise, diet, stress, etc.–her problems would most certainly disappear. And that is exactly what the internist also suggested when I referred Elaine to him because of my concern about her chest pain. The internist did a stress ECG and concluded that the chest pain was really related to her heartburn and her problems were manageable if she would just be willing to address her life-style. So in the meantime she takes antidepressant pills, pills for her heartburn, and, because her joints bother her so much, she takes antiarthritic medication on occasion–in spite of the fact that these pills can aggravate her gut.

I know her relationship with her husband isn't good. I know that occasionally he threatens her. On the most recent visit she said: "I'm just trying to hang in there for one more year and then I plan to get a divorce. Lisa (her daughter) has just one more year before she finishes her degree and then it won't matter if he doesn't support us financially. But it's scary. Lately he's been worse and partly it's because he's been home more. Money really isn't an issue for us. We have significant property, but he's so stingy. He doesn't want to support Lisa, but so far he has. I know if I leave him that will be the end of the money. With the way things drag out in court it could be years before a settlement. The psychologist I saw years ago told me he didn't think my husband was the violent type. He thought he just liked to threaten, but I'm not so sure. Lisa and I both put locks on our bedroom doors recently. Generally when he's at home I just keep myself locked in the room. I talk with my kids about where and how I'll live when I leave him. We all seem to think that I'll need to live close to one of them–otherwise it's just too frightening.

Elaine's presence fully registered on me during that visit. Her body hidden under a shapeless dress. Her blue eyes framed by grey permed hair seemed lost in tears. Her never-ending questions and concerns created a sense of doom in my office.

I gave Elaine more pills. I knew that nagging at her to lose weight was ineffective. Furthermore, I suspected that food represented her main comfort in life.

Besides, who was I anyway to simply suggest that her solutions were easy–that this was just a matter of Elaine's life-style?

Elaine Sanders

Elaine has four children. Panic attacks. Headaches. Stomach pains. I asked questions. We talked. She got counseling. He agreed to get counselling. The family went for counseling. The oldest daughter threatened to leave. He stopped hitting the daughter. Then he started threatening Elaine again. She arranged to leave. He said he would try again. They went for counseling. Sometimes she took antidepressants. Sometimes her headaches stopped and sometimes the stomach pains eased up, but more often than not Elaine experienced health problems.

She said: "Sometimes I feel so stupid that I can't figure this out. Sometimes I feel like he just wants to be seen with me. I feel like I'm on a roller coaster. I feel so vulnerable. I feel so crazy. Sometimes when I'm alone I feel like me, and then I feel better. But when I'm with him I'm confused. He's always putting me down. Sometimes it's like I'm watching myself. I know when I'm there and when I'm not. He's jealous of me. Possesive. Sometimes I feel so tired."

But finally after 18 years she and the three children moved out. The oldest daughter had already left home. Elaine wondered why she had stayed so long. Elaine wondered, now that she had moved out, if she would feel better.

I wondered about the pain problems these women experienced. Their pain problems could not be reduced to simple "diagnosis and cure" solutions. Their pain probems inevitably were complex and often the pain story was a story of relationship struggle. And in time, I wondered why we rarely value the way women struggle to keep relationships alive, the way women struggle to understand that we do not live in isolation, the way women struggle against a culture that condemns us when we leave our husbands, a culture that condemns us when we try to stay, a culture that tells us we are codependent when we try to help him, a culture that tells us over and over that we mothers and wives have failed, and keeps asking us when he hurts us and our sons and daughters "why in God's name don't you just leave him?" What would happen if we all just left him?

Chapter 11

Janet:
Stop Talking

> She is dressed in a fairly pricey cotton dress and light blue summer coat, her hair short and swept back and upwards. At this moment she hates it all, this external self who is at such variance with whatever or whoever remains inside the glossy painted shell. If anything remains. Her remains.
>
> –Margaret Laurence, *The Diviners*

JANET'S STORY

Sometimes I'm prepared for the "Kleenex moment" and at other times it catches me completely off guard. On that day I felt unprepared.

Janet looked at me, her brown eyes filled with anguish. She always seemed like such an efficient, organized, and rather normal person, so the pained look caught my attention.

"I really wonder if maybe it's me that's crazy," she said, and then began sobbing. I had to quickly tune in.

I had known Janet for 10 years. Her health problems had been straightforward. I cared for her during her most recent pregnancy, and apart from her occasional tension headaches and neck pain she coped well.

Sometimes I think I envied her. She had one of those bodies that always seemed the right size–not too thin and not too fat. Her hair had that natural look–blond-brown with soft curls–that you see in shampoo adds. Her clothes always looked comfortable but just fashionable enough for her job as a teacher. She always seemed so together.

"What's happened?"

"It's complicated," she continued. "I know my marriage, job, and kids all seem okay on the outside, but everything's falling apart. And my head and neck are starting to kill me again. I'm tired. I just can't understand Don anymore and I'm not sure I've got the energy left to try."

I had met Don on a few occasions when he came in with the children (a son and a daughter–ages eight and thirteen), so I felt at least somewhat acquainted with him. It seemed difficult to understand her dilemma. Don appeared to be a caring parent and husband. I knew his job as a lawyer kept him busy, but their family unit had always seemed to function.

"I'm not sleeping and I just can't concentrate anymore. I keep thinking I've got to leave Don. He says I'm crazy and I'm starting to think he's right." She began to sob uncontrollably.

I waited.

"I'm sorry," she said.

"You don't need to apologize, Janet. Things don't seem to be going very well."

"You've got that right."

"Anyway," she said, as she looked up and reached for the Kleenex, "'I need help. Maybe I've got some terrible disease–oh–I don't know–I think I just need to talk to someone. I'm sure it's marriage counseling we need, but Don doesn't want to go that route so I'm going alone. I told him I felt it was time to find out how fundamentally crazy I really am."

"Okay, Janet," I said, "let's take this a step at a time."

The level of her depression concerned me. I needed to determine her suicide risk but that didn't seem to be an issue. I suggested she take a few days off just to get some relief from the anguish but she couldn't see that as an option with her job commitments. We talked about counselors, their various approaches and fees, etc.

I suggested she start taking antidepressants. She readily agreed. I gave her some pills to get started and she agreed to return in two weeks. I hoped by then she would have at least connected with a therapist and that the medication would be having some effect. At the moment she looked too tired and disorganized for any rational thought. She had a complete checkup only two months ago, but I decided to order a thyroid test and hemoglobin. I couldn't help but wonder what was really going on but with Janet's level of exhaustion, extensive questioning at the moment seemed inappropriate and futile. I advised her to book for a longer appointment with the next visit. I wanted to address–in a more complete fashion–her physical concerns as well as the depression.

Two Weeks Later

Janet returned. She didn't look rested, but the anguish had left her face. "I've started the counseling," she volunteered. "I'm not expecting miracles, but hopefully I'll be able to sort some of this mess out."

"Are you sleeping any better?"

"That's really improved," she continued, "so I presume I should stay on the pills."

I agreed and adjusted the dosage.

"My headaches seem to have decreased," she continued, "but my neck really bugs me."

We started talking about her neck, but without realizing what happened we were on the topic of Don. She seemed to need to ventilate. "It's crazy. I feel okay at work, but the minute I step into the house it's as if I'm a different person. I'm competent at my job, but at home it's like I'm not capable of any decisions. He criticizes me for the smallest problems. From his perspective I do very little right. And when it's not right, watch out. His anger scares me, although he's never hit me. I know I'm always trying to prevent those rages of his, but I can never get it right." She paused and then continued. "That's not true come to think of it. Sometimes he seems okay. Like I've figured out how to really take care of him and then for some reason all hell breaks loose. Sometimes he seems so possessive and jealous of me." She sighed. I nodded. I encouraged her to continue therapy. I tried to get her to focus on any behavioral patterns she could address.

I reviewed the lab tests and did a physical check to satisfy her and myself that the headaches and neck pain were part of a muscle tension problem.

Because of the neck pain and headaches, I encouraged her to take time to get some physiotherapy. She had excuses for avoiding therapy–interferes with the kids' schedule, who will make supper, he'll be frustrated, etc.

I challenged her with some of this thinking. "So what if he gets angry? He doesn't hit you." (That issue can be pretty tricky and I'm careful how I approach the real risk of violence in the lives of many women). "He's entitled to his anger and frustration. You're going to need to take responsibility for your stuff and move out of the blaming mode," I suggested.

"Easier said then done," she commented.

We agreed she would see me once a month while she continued on the antidepressants. I encouraged exercise and sensible eating behavior.

Janet left with a commitment to addressing some of the issues. She agreed to return in a month.

I thought about how often I observed this pattern in my office. The productive, efficient public woman in contrast to the compliant private woman. How come? And of course, in Janet's situation I realized that I knew a lot about her and her background because I cared for her mother and two sisters as well. I understood that she came from one of those perfect families where no one argued. I knew that Janet's difficulty expressing herself in her marriage reflected this pattern of compliance she had learned while growing up, yet I suspected that there were cultural issues as well. Why? Because I see far too many women struggling in relationships, and so often they're depressed and in some sort of physical pain.

Six Months Later

Janet continued therapy and eventually progressed to a group program. She continued her medication. Her depression and anxiety fluctuated dramatically at times. Her moments of despair gradually lessened and I perceived her moving toward taking greater responsibility for her own needs.

Her physical pain and fatigue markedly decreased when she joined a dance class. She described it this way.

"I took ballet lessons when I was a kid. I remember that I loved the movement and that physical feeling. I had forgotten all of that. Now, in this class sometimes my body feels so alive. It's as if all of my emotions–sadness, anger, pain, joy, and happiness–can be felt in my toes, my fingers, my face, and my everything."

She adjusted her schedule, much to her husbands' frustration. At times she described her emerging anger. She said, "It seems as I find my space for direct anger I'm less controlled by his. I see so often that his anger has mostly to do with his stuff–not just me. That's a relief. I know I'm not crazy."

One Year Later

About a year after she had started therapy, Janet returned looking more rested and peaceful than I had ever seen her. "So, what's new?"

"Lots," she said. "Do you have a few minutes?"

Fortunately, I wasn't behind.

"I've taken such a big step and I want to tell you about it."

"Go ahead, I'm listening,"

She continued.

"The group business had been going rather slowly and I realized it had to do with me. I knew I needed to work harder. Anyway, we negotiate with the therapist for extra time and finally I decided to address that stuck feeling. It's crazy. I'm 41 years old. I know it's not about pleasing my parents, my husband, or anyone else, and yet that seemed to be exactly where I sat. You know–I'm not thin enough. My work isn't good enough. I'm a lousy mother. It's my fault my husband isn't happy, and on and on. The therapist kept trying to get me to take responsibility. It's not easy. Our culture gives women so many mixed messages. Be responsible but don't let anyone know how capable you really are. Be seductive and sexy but don't be strong. It's all fine and wonderful to say that I should be the judge of my life, but where is my life anyway? Have I ever really had any say in this? The anguish had become too much. I had to address this stuff."

I nodded as she continued.

"We do little drama scenarios in group and the therapist thought it would be useful to reenact my parent issue. I agreed, although in comparison to the abuse and awful stuff that other group members experienced my dilemmas seemed trivial."

She described the following scene.

"So, we sat in a circle–the therapist across from me, two members became the imaginary father and mother. At first "the parents" stood in front of me–beside each other. Somehow that didn't seem right. Finally the therapist placed the father behind the mother with his hand on her shoulder and suddenly it clicked. That seemed right. What are the parents doing, she kept asking me. That wasn't easy. No, they didn't hurt me, I told the therapist. No one hit in our house. So she kept questioning me about what happened. What were your parents saying, she asked me."

I could picture Janet's scene as she continued.

Janet said: "Then it came to me. I thought–Janet stop talking, stop talking, stop talking. That's it, I told the therapist. I couldn't talk. There was no point in talking–I wasn't heard–so I stopped talking." Janet looked intensely at me and continued, "The therapist then told the imaginary parents to play that scene. So the mother started saying as she looked at me 'Janet stop talking, stop talking, stop talking,' and the imaginary father nodded and nodded and smiled and agreed."

Janet's story mesmerized me and I began filling the details in my head as Janet finished her story. Janet–on the floor with her hand over her head. Head bowed low. The mother shaking her finger at Janet and saying loudly, "stop talking, stop talking, stop talking." I don't want to hear that ever again.

I could see the therapist encouraging Janet to respond to her parents as Janet struggled to get her head up. The force from her parents seemed too great. And then finally she got onto her knees, put her hand out, and gasped, "Mom–Dad–I can talk. I have my voice and you cannot take it from me ever again."

I could see the therapist as she intervened for Janet and cautioned the imaginary parents to move back into the circle. I could see Janet collapsed on the floor in pain and agony. And then the therapist waits until Janet raises her head and reaches for the person next to her. Janet looks at all members in the group and I imagine her saying, "no one can ever stop my voice again."

I realized Janet had finished her story. Her face blurred in front of me. I sensed her power and strength.

Our eyes met and we smiled tears of joy.

"You're on the way, Janet–great work."

I continue to see bits and pieces of Janet's life. Sometimes her voice fades to a mere whisper as she continues her journey, and at other times her voice comes through loud and clear. She no longer needs antidepressants. Her headaches still occur, but no longer dominate her life. Her search for meaning and connection continue.

Now, with Janet seeing her way clearer, I can't help but wonder about other women who are depressed and why it is that twice as many women as men are depressed in the first place? Or why I keep seeing so many women with physical pain where depression is clearly a big part of the picture. When I read standard medical textbooks and listen to the "experts" on the topic of depression, so often it sounds like depression is just an intrapsychic issue–you know, something that just has to do with you. So, of course, you just need pills–and new antidepressant pills are manufactured regularly. It seems there is just a chemical imbalance–we all may just need Prozac or you just need to become more self-sufficient or something like that. But that doesn't seem to be what I hear in my office. It's unusual when I think about it to even identify depression in any woman without at the same time hearing a story of relationship pain and struggle of some sort. In thinking about women's depression, inevitably I think about the energy required for women to be passive and silent. Depression is both individual and social. Depression combines the personal and the political. One cannot heal the self in isolation and of course I see that over and over again. It's interesting for me to read what women psychologists are writing about the importance of relational development for women. It's a relief that human reality does not have to just reflect the self-contained autonomous male perspective. I can begin to value the way women struggle in relationships. It seems that I can move in a direction that is supportive rather than a direction that again defines the women as defective and in need of fixing. And so, I too struggle with the complexity of physical pain, depression, and relationship issues that are daily concerns in my office.

Chapter 12

Laura: Another Roadblock

> She reached for the stack of files, his fingers sliding over hers as he handed them to her. Surprised, she looked up to his deliberate eyes on her face. And an hour later, the office deserted, was less surprised to feel those same cool, narrow fingers on the back of her neck, lifting her hair and turning her face upwards.
>
> –Aritha van Herk, *Judith*

LAURA'S STORY

"I need to get this pain thing figured out," Laura said. "I've been to several doctors, and specialists as well. It's just that they can't seem to figure it out. And it's causing a problem for me. It bothers me. Why do I have days where I feel okay and then some days the pain in my gut–stomach–or somewhere down there creates a real problem for me?"

"Ummm, I don't know Laura, but I think we should start from the beginning of the story and take things a step at a time. And I'd like to get your past records, because there is no point in subjecting you to unnecessary tests," I responded.

This was Laura's first visit. I noticed from the chart that Laura was 28. Immediately, I sensed her frustration and almost despair. She looked sad. Her average-looking body occupied the chair in a somewhat resigned manner. I can't really remember anything else about her that day. Her clothes, makeup, and hair seemed ordinary–not meant to attract unnecessary attention. Everything about her seemed to say–look, no one else could help me, I really don't expect much from you.

So I proceeded in my usual fashion. I sensed hidden pieces somewhere in the story.

"So, are you in pain right now?"

"No. That's what bugs me. Wouldn't you know it? Today I'm fine."

"Okay," I said, "then I'll just take some history and get you to book for a longer appointment on your next visit. And let's get this form signed so that we can get records."

I decided to concentrate on the history of the pain problem and her past medical history, knowing that on the next visit I could complete the information.

"So, tell me about the pain?"

"It started several years ago. I can't remember for sure but sometime in my early twenties. At first I was just aware of an occasional cramping feeling. Sometimes I thought it was just related to my periods, but then other times it didn't seem to have anything to do with that. Sometimes I would feel incredibly bloated. And then I would have episodes of diarrhea and sometimes I'm incredibly constipated."

"Ummmm. Ever any blood in your stools?"

"No, nothing like that. And they took a bunch of stool samples. I don't want to have to do that again. They couldn't find anything wrong. I had that barium enema test, too, and I don't want that again. They sent me to a specialist and I had that other test–you know," she hesitated. "A sigmoidoscopy," I said. "Yes, that's it. And I don't want that again either."

"Ummmm, so your gut's been checked out."

"You could say that, but that's not all. Sometimes my pain seems to have more to do with my periods–my uterus and ovary stuff. Anyway–they checked that out too. I had one of those tests where they make the incision around the belly-button–you know," she hesitated again. "Oh, you had a laparoscopy." I said. "Yes, that's it. So you see I've had lots of tests and they can't find anything wrong, but I still have pain. That's what is so frustrating. Something has to be wrong."

"Yes, this sounds frustrating and I certainly don't want to repeat any tests unless we think it necessary. My only suggestion for now is to please keep a record of the pain–when it happens, what you've eaten, etc. Make another appointment and next visit we'll talk more and I'll check you over. I don't suppose I'll have any magic, but perhaps we can try to make some sense of this pain problem."

"So what do you think? Am I crazy or something? How can I have this pain and all those tests be normal? I'm so tired of being told that everything is okay when obviously it isn't."

"No, I'm sure you're not crazy, Laura. But when it comes to pain problems I think we often try to find simple answers when there just aren't any. So my approach is that you and I together will try to make some sense of this."

"What do you mean–you and I together? What am I supposed to do?"

"To be honest, I'm not completely sure, but it just seems that we both better get thinking, because trying to find the answer just with tests hasn't worked."

"That's vague. But I'll keep track of that stuff and if I get any terrible pains before my next visit can I come back sooner?"

"Of course."

And Laura left.

I knew this seemed vague. But it is vague. No one understands chronic pain problems. And look what happens when we try to solve chronic pain problems in a simple fashion. People get investigated to death by everyone. Patients are left feeling worse–crazy. So even if sometimes I don't really understand this process, I'm at least trying to shift into another approach and another way to understand the pain.

Laura's records arrived a few weeks later. Not too surprising. Laparoscopy and pelvic ultrasound scan–normal. Barium enema, sigmoidoscopy, and stool cultures–normal. She even had a cystoscopy, a procedure where the doctor puts a scope into the bladder and looks. This too was normal, as was her intravenous pyelogram, which is a test to check the kidneys. Her most recent pap test had been over a year ago, so at least there was something left for me to do!

Three Weeks Later

Laura arrived looking anxious. "Did you get my records?"

"Yes, and I've had some time to look them over. I see you've had quite a bit of investigation."

"So, what do you think?"

"I think, Laura, that we should proceed as planned. Let me ask more questions, then I'll do the physical exam and we'll talk about what all of this means."

"Okay."

"So, did you keep track of the pain stuff?"

"Yes, the last few weeks haven't been too bad, but I had two days with bad cramps in my gut. I don't think it's related to anything I eat, although maybe some vegetables do bother me. It seems as if the afternoons are more of a problem. And I'm wondering about coffee. I don't drink much, but on one of the days I had three extra cups because I was in a meeting, and I don't know if that was the issue–it's hard to say because the meeting was frustrating in itself."

"Ummm. So no obvious patterns."

"Not really."

I reviewed her previous investigations and made sure she understood the reason for the test and what the test could exclude when the test was normal. She found some of this information interesting because it seemed that with some of the tests she had not really understood why the test was done.

I continued with questions about the family and social history.

"Laura, I ask many questions about the family you grew up in and your present family, so just try to answer the questions and realize that this is standard information I get from everyone."

She nodded.

"Let's start with your parents. Are they healthy?"

"Oh–I don't know about my father. My parents separated when I was five and my mother never talks about him and I've never met him."

"Umm."

"So–about your mother."

"Oh, yes, she's healthy. Nothing wrong with her."

"And what about her parents?"

"I think her mother died of lung cancer and I'm not sure about her father. He died before I was born."

"And do you have siblings?"

"No–it was just me. And my mother never remarried. So I grew up with just Mom."

"Any family history of breast cancer, arthritis, or heart disease?"

"To tell you the honest truth, I wouldn't know. I'm not sure if I even have any other relatives. I think I met some cousins once, but that was a long time ago. My mother's a bit different. She never had anything to do with relatives."

"Ummm. Sounds like you and your mother were a bit isolated while you were growing up."

"Yes, you could say that."

And then we talked more about her childhood. She spent a great deal of time with her mother. She seemed to be her mother's companion. But also her mother seemed to expect a great deal from her. And when questioned about abuse she completely denied that as an issue and yet clearly stated that her mother was exacting and regularly hit her to get compliance. She spoke about her obvious pain with respect to her mother. Her mother appeared to be successful in her business but probably not so successful in her personal life. The fact that she had no contact with her father and no desire to meet him was something that she blamed her mother for. She had recalled a few times when she had conversations with her mother about her father and she thought that maybe he did have an alcohol problem–and her mother had implied that he had been in jail once.

"So, do you see your mother much now?"

"Oh, I visit occasionally but it's so frustrating. My mother doesn't approve of me in too many ways. She doesn't like my boyfriend, she thinks my job isn't good enough, and in general I guess she somehow views me as a failure–not too surprising I find the visits stressful."

"So have you ever talked to anyone about this–you know–a counselor?"

"Not really. There's not much you can do about the past."

"That's true, but sometimes talking about these things can help us see them clearer, so that these experiences don't keep weighing us down. You know, in listening to you I sense that there's a part of you that feels sort of hopeless yourself–that is, that you almost believe your mother that you're somehow a failure."

"Well, that's sort of true and I know at my job I try so hard to please my boss and it never works. Even sometimes I see the same thing with my boyfriend. I don't want to lose him. So I try hard–oh, sometimes everything seems hopeless."

"Ummmm – we'll talk more about that."

And then she told me more about her present situations. Her job as an executive secretary was a job she liked, but there was no question that she experienced daily stress. The stress inevitably revolved around the boss. There wasn't any obvious sexual harassment. Laura had clearly removed his hands once and let him know to never do that again. But Laura experienced continual episodes that left her off balance–last minute demands, inappropriate remarks in front of other staff, at times seeming to withhold important information from her and then at the last minute making her look like she wasn't prepared at meetings, things she just couldn't put her fingers on, things that often left her confused.

Her relationship with her boyfriend worked fairly well, and at the moment she hoped he wouldn't push her for any commitments. She felt she needed him, but was scared of closeness and had managed a relationship with convenient distance.

Questions about other potential health issues were all negative responses. If she could just solve this cramping abdominal pain she would be healthy.

I proceeded to the physical examination. I checked her carefully. I did her pap test and took cultures. Her examination was normal.

I left the room while Laura dressed and quickly caught up with a few other patients. I returned to the room for further discussion with Laura.

"So, what do you think?"

"Okay–let's sum this up," I said. "You have a story of abdominal pain. On your physical examination I can see no obvious problem. I've taken your pap test and cultures, but I really expect them to be normal. In reviewing your investigations many problems have been ruled out, and I can safely say that I don't think you have any serious or life-threatening sort of problem. Rather, your story and the tests are compatible with a diagnosis of irritable bowel syndrome."

"What's that? Is that like colitis?"

"Well, sometimes people do refer to it that way, but colitis really isn't a good term, because people can for instance have ulcerative colitis, which is a very difficult disease, and you certainly don't have that."

"Well, this seems a bit weird to me. Those other doctors told me I had something just like you said. What was that again?"

"I think you have irritable bowel syndrome."

"So let's get rid of it."

"That's where the difficulty comes in. This really isn't a pain problem that is readily fixed. Rather, it is something that you likely will always be prone to. But there are things that can help you."

"Like what?"

"Well, there's no question but that adding fiber to your diet helps. You can do this by just simply adding raw bran that you find in the grocery store or you can buy any number of products in the drugstore that are meant to add bulk to your diet."

"Well, that's what those other doctors told me already."

"So did you try that?"

"Well, yes, but not for very long. It didn't really seem to work, and I don't really get this. I don't want to take something for life. I want to get this problem figured out."

"But that's the point, Laura. The problem is figured out as best as we doctors know how to figure it out, and from here on it's sort of up to you."

"No one ever said that before."

"Well, I guess that's what I'm saying. I'd like you to try to increase the bulk in your diet consistently for a month. Also, it's my observation that people who exercise regularly have less problem with this bloating-cramping thing."

Laura looked less than convinced, but agreed to try some changes for a month and then she would return. I told her I'd call if the pap and cultures showed any problem.

Accepting a chronic pain problem seems to be difficult for doctors and patients alike. What is it about our culture that perpetuates this notion–that there is an easy solution to complex pain problems (an easy solution to everything really), that life must be easy, that technology can solve everything, that life cannot be difficult. What is it that makes it so difficult for any of us to accept uncertainty? I suppose it's about fear to a certain extent. Fear that there is something terribly wrong, fear that the doctor missed something, and the doctor certain that there is just one more test that will find the answer. And we're all afraid–afraid of something–afraid–"What if this pain is about something that I might die from?" Or, if I'm the doctor, "What if I forgot that crucial test?" Yes–afraid about this thing that says, "Eventually we all die–and when we all die, we die alone." But of course this seems ridiculous–seeing the doctor about pain in the gut doesn't have anything to do with this.

One Month Later

Laura returned. "I think maybe the fiber helps but I'm not sure. Actually I had sort of an awful time at my mother's last week. That's what's really bothering me."

"So what happened?"

"My mother is on my case. She doesn't like my boyfriend. I think I see now that she really doesn't like men. I guess she's never had a relationship that worked. Anyway–she started in on me. My gut really acted up when I was there."

And then she suddenly stopped.

She put her hands to her throat. "I feel like I'm choking–I'm nauseated."

Her body went forward on the chair. She put her hands over her eyes. "This feels so awful."

Silence.

"Laura, I can see this hurts."

"Oh, I'm sorry. It's just that I realized this time when I was home how suffocated I felt." And she looked up with eyes filled with tears.

"Maybe I should talk to that counselor you were talking about. I can't stand this feeling." Her hands wrapped around her body–seeming to need to hold herself together.

"Yes, I think it would be a good idea. You could benefit from some support and some way to resolve and understand some of this stuff."

We talked more. Laura agreed to see the counselor and I suggested she return in a month or so. Her gut pain was still a big issue.

One Year Later

"Laura. So how are you?"

"Well, a lot has changed. I went to the counselor. It helped. At least I can see how some of my problems fit together. And I've resolved so much of that stuff with my mother. It's not that we have a close relationship but at least I can see how her struggles to get through life have affected me and now I know it's up to me to set my own agenda. And I even have a better handle on the gut stuff. I have pain and cramps still but I don't worry like I used to. I guess I really thought there was something terrible wrong with me. And I'm finding ways to avoid some of the things that set the gut off–I've stopped coffee completely–things like that and I still take that fiber stuff. But that's not why I'm here."

"So what are we doing today?"

"It's my job. I'm going crazy. With the counseling I feel like I'm really getting a handle on things. I can see now how my boss is sort of just like my mother and how I get sucked into so much garbage. Just when I'm thinking that I'm getting clearer I experience something crazy at work–it feels like another roadblock. I'm sick of roadblocks. What I want is a week away from my job. I plan to think things through. Either I get a handle on this job problem or I'm going to quit. I'm starting to see how often my gut acts up after one of those crazy scenarios with the boss. And either he's getting worse or I'm seeing through his tricks easier. I'm not sure which. Anyway, my health is too important to ignore."

"Ummmm. You've really taken some steps, Laura."

She nodded.

"Sure–take a week off and think it through. But be sure to return and let me know what you're up to. I may need to fill forms out or something for you, so I have to understand what's happening."

We talked more. We talked about roadblocks.

"What's frustrating for me is that sometimes I feel it's just me. You know. I'm crazy. But then I know it isn't just me. I found out that the last woman at this job left for health reasons. I'm thinking I have to go to the man above my boss. I don't know if it'll do any good but it's the only route I can see. What bugs me is that this stuff is so subtle. If he were just pawing all over me I could get the attention of the committee on sexual harassment and get everyone's support immediately. But that's not it. It's the way he keeps putting me down, keeps me off balance, and in general seems to go out of his way to irritate me. Sometimes I feel like he plays games with me just like I'm his wife or something."

And I talked to Laura about my observations in my office. The fact that I saw many women struggling with roadblocks in their jobs; the fact that many women's health problems were aggravated by these subtle and sometimes not so subtle problems at work. The fact that I didn't think in many cases that these problems were really personal issues as much as cultural issues. Laura left.

I thought about how often I heard about roadblocks. Just when a woman feels as if she's getting things figured out she faces that block of cement in front of her at the job. So often the questions the women raised were: "Is it just me? Or is this about other women too? Does he just do this to me? How much do men experience this at work?" And so often this stress translates into health issues for women–headaches, irritable bowel syndrome, depression, neck pains. Often it seemed that the way I helped these women was to point this out: "No, it's not about just you. No, your boss isn't just picking on you personally. It's about something else. It's about women and the way women are not heard. It's about the way women at work feel isolated and unable to proceed clearly. It's about sexual harassment, only this form is so subtle."

Two Years Later

"Laura. So what's happening?"

"Oh, I just need to get more birth control pills today. I know you don't have time for the pap now. I've booked for that later."

"You look great, Laura," I commented. She looked energetic. She smiled. Her hair shone. Her brown eyes sparkled.

"Gee–do I look that different?"

"Yes, you do."

"Well, I made some changes. You remember that job?"

"Of course I do."

"Well, I went to the man above my boss and things did improve for a while. But then I could see the pattern recurring. And in the meantime, I did more talking with a friend. You won't believe this, but we've started a business together. It's going slow, but it sure feels good to know where you're at. And at least with Arlene I can agree, disagree, and together we struggle. None of that bullshit game-playing stuff."

"Wow–just look at you."

Laura laughed and beamed.

"And my poor old gut. To think what I went through trying to get it sorted out. Yes, it's amazing. I still get cramps, but it's in perspective now. And even though I have incredible stress with this new business it's a different kind of stress. It's stress that I've created. Not stress that someone else controls."

"Wow–you sure see things clearer today."

"You've got that right."

And Laura left.

Later, I thought about other women similar to Laura–Tara, Shelly, Nancy, and Sylvia. They experienced other variations of the theme of roadblocks.

Tara's Roadblock

She spent a good year struggling after the sexual assault. The assault occurred in her house. The neighbor was drunk. She let him in before she realized that. She fought him off and called the police. Not too surprisingly, the court case and the trauma of it all affected her profoundly. Not too surprisingly, she struggled with panic attacks and headaches. Not too surprisingly, she didn't get the promotion she had hoped for that year. She just didn't have the energy to struggle with that too. Not too surprisingly, it all felt like a roadblock.

Shelly's Roadblock

She didn't tell many people about her roadblock. When her stomach pains escalated I asked many questions. Finally she talked. "I don't know how I let myself get involved with that professor at college. I should have know better. But I did. We had an affair. And of course it ended badly. Now, I think the only way I can get on with things is to try to get into another school. I think I've probably lost a year's worth of work. How could I have been so stupid?" Shelly didn't really view this as a roadblock. She viewed it completely as her problem.

It's tough for women–when you're young–and someone finally seems to notice you–to think that maybe you have ideas that are worth listening to–it's tough to get all the power stuff figured out at the same time.

Nancy's Roadblock

When her colleague at work sexually harassed her she stopped him immediately. She reported him. Then she spent a year struggling with what that meant. When her headaches escalated she had a good handle on the problem. On one occasion she said to me: "Just think how much more I could have accomplished this year if it wasn't for all that garbage?" She knew about roadblocks and knew how to push them out of the way. It's just that it takes so damn much energy.

Sylvia's Roadblock

When Sylvia expressed concern that day about her problems with stress and neck pain she said: "What really bugs me is that I know that this stress at the job is a big part of my health problem. I really wanted to get the vice-principal job. I know there are many women teachers who don't want administrative positions. But I do. When they gave the job to a male colleague with five years less experience it really bugged me. I helped him cope with some pretty basic stuff this past year. Sometimes I feel so angry, but then the old self-doubt stuff surfaces–well maybe I'm not competent for the job–but then I know that's just not true. How can I fight the system when it seems that there is no one in a position of power who is on my side?"

Other Roadblocks

And, of course, there are endless variations on the roadblock and ill-health theme–"I thought dating him would be okay. I couldn't believe how he forced himself on me and now the panic attacks won't go away. I don't want to see that doctor again. I don't know why he always pushes his body against mine when it seems so unnecessary–maybe it's my imagination but I never want to go back there again."

But at least women can begin to see that there are roadblocks everywhere and that these roadblocks aren't about them personally. Roadblocks are about power and control–and about a system that has given power to men and where men far too often continue to define the power that women cannot have and continue to define a role for women that is for the convenience of men. But of course what if Laura talks to Nancy, and Nancy talks to Shelly, and Shelly talks to Tara, and Tara talks to Sylvia, and they all realize it's not about them personally? I sense that far too often, in spite of everything we think we know, that Laura, Nancy, Shelly, Tara, and Sylvia don't talk that much about personal roadblocks. Far too often, these women see their roadblocks as personal issues–personal failures and hence something to keep to themselves; something that is so painful; something to hide. After all, everywhere about them women do seem to be succeeding in many ways and it is women who may reinforce the notion that, "look, it is about you personally because after all, look, I've succeeded."

But maybe–just maybe–the roadblocks won't seem so big if together Laura, Tara, Shelly, Nancy, and Sylvia start talking, start being more honest, start clearly defining roadblocks, and then start collecting the equipment needed to push the roadblocks out of the way. Perhaps then Laura, Tara, Shelly, Nancy, and Sylvia can begin to define a new system–a system where they have a say, where they are heard, where they can define what it's all about for them.

Chapter 13

Ellen: Lost Voices Everywhere

> By sharing reactions and solutions, whether about child-rearing, domestic problems, or weight reduction, by being given the opportunity to talk things over with a sympathetic, nonjudgmental person with similar experiences, a woman can begin to hear that maybe she is not such an incompetent, a dummy, or an oddity. She has experience that may be valuable to others; she, too, can know things.
>
> –Belenky et al., *Women's Ways of Knowing*

I glanced at my watch as I opened the door to the examining room. On time. Just one more patient to see and I would be finished for the morning. I didn't want to be late for lunch. I had just met Ellen a few months ago at a conference on women's health. We shared so many ideas. The connection had been instant. I looked forward to more conversation with her. Ellen and I were similar ages and seemed to be at similar points in our lives.

"One?" the hostess questioned. "No, there will be two of us," I said as I quickly glanced about the restaurant, realizing that Ellen hadn't arrived.

"May I bring you something to drink?"

"Yes, tea please," I said to the waitress who already looked frazzled.

And then I saw Ellen. She sat down quickly and muttered, "Tax time, we're so busy."

"Don't remind me," I laughed.

Sometimes I thought Ellen's job as an accountant had distinct advantages, but today I sensed I should stick to people and not numbers. We scanned menus. The waitress arrived and rattled off the specials.

"Are you ready to order?"

"Yes." We responded simultaneously.

"I'll have the stir-fry thing you described," I said immediately and Ellen ordered the sandwich special.

We both were acutely aware of the limited time.

"So–how are things?"

"Job is crazy right now." And then Ellen took a deep breath and seemed to relax. "But I want to tell you about my weekend with my daughter. I mentioned her, didn't I?"

"Yes–Aleta–isn't that her name? And isn't she in university?"

"Yes. That's her."

Ellen filled me in on a weekend that sounded wonderful to me. Of course daughters aren't perfect, but Ellen and her daughter seemed to be moving into a nice adult relationship. Ellen talked about daughters in general and how she hoped that they would see things sooner.

"Aleta isn't sure what her major will be. Sometimes I feel concerned. On one hand I want her to be practical. The job market is so crazy these days. On the other hand I hope that she can have an opportunity to just–you know–expand her mind."

"Ummm, university days should certainly have some of that," I responded.

"Aleta is taking a psychology course and we had an amazing conversation about the book *Women's Ways of Knowing*. She's been reading it for one of her classes–do you know that book?"

"Yes, I do. That's funny," I said. "I just had a conversation with my sister about that book. She's in education. I couldn't believe how we both thought alike in so many areas, and she's a sister I always thought I was so different from."

We both smiled.

"It's the part of the book where they talk about subjective knowledge that I really understood," I said. "I've struggled so much to believe what I know I see and feel and then the struggle to somehow make sense of my own ideas while still so influenced by the notion that knowledge or truth is something out there–something that someone else figures out."

"Yes, I know what you mean. Aleta and I talked about that a lot."

The waitress interrupted our thoughts as she carefully placed plates on the table. "Can I get you anything else?" she said.

We both shook our heads.

I glanced at my watch again.

"Can't you stop looking at your watch?" Ellen teased me.

"No," I laughed. "Look–this conversation is just getting started and it's already twelve thirty!"

"I have an idea. Next time let's have dinner. I'm feeling pressured too."

We quickly inhaled some food.

"But back to that inner voice and knowledge stuff," Ellen said while swallowing. "Sometimes at work I experience something that feels like what we're talking about only it's different. It's what seems to happen when I'm discussing accounting problems–sometimes I feel like I'll say something and then I wonder if anyone heard me. You know I'm the only female accountant in our firm. But what bugs me is–a male says something–and in many cases he will be junior to me–and then I sense he is heard but I'm not. I know it's crazy. But that's just it. Is it crazy? Is it my imagination or is this experience real? Or am I just paranoid?"

"Wow," I said. "Do you realize how close those words are to what my sister said about her experience in her academic world?"

"Really?"

"Uh, uh!"

"You know this is on the same lines as all that's being written about men and women in conversation. We speak different languages, except that it seems women can learn men's language to survive if they need to," I continued.

"Yes, I've heard that too. I think that's what I struggle with. How to be heard? And then the feeling, though, that I have to suppress so much of what I see and how I approach things in order to be heard. And then I feel less real. Doesn't this sound crazy?" Ellen paused and then continued. "And then occasionally I have these experiences–one on one–with a male colleague, where I'm left feeling incredibly put down but where I know if I try to address the issues I'll look like another sensitive whiny female. It's so irritating. I'm seriously wondering if maybe I should look elsewhere to work. Perhaps even work on my own. Even if I made less money, perhaps it would be worth it–this torture stuff would stop. Wow–this is nuts!"

"Are you kidding? It's a relief for me to hear you say this stuff."

I motioned for the waitress. "Could I have more hot water, please?"

"I struggle with this stuff in every aspect of my life but I'm acutely aware of two separate things," I said. "With my patients, many of whom are female, I'm aware of how easy it is for me to slip into some sort of mode that is the expert thing–the person with knowledge thing–that I'm just starting to see really limits my ability to be in conversation, particularly with women. I think it has to do with being in a male-dominated profession and learning the male way of being in the world, so to speak. And of course I need to have that sense of identity as a doctor to function, or so I think. But–then I feel a constriction. And when in conversation with colleagues I experience something else. When I have different ideas or challenge the usual medical interpretation I find myself off balance. I find myself asking the same questions you ask. Am I crazy? Can I believe what I see and feel, or is what I am experiencing untrustworthy? Why do I sometimes feel so silenced with my ideas?"

"I can't believe you just said all of that."

Ellen and I were both lost in thought and I noticed that we pushed food around on our plates methodically.

"That reminds me," Ellen said, "about a few of my visits with doctors years ago. You remember I mentioned that abuse stuff when we talked at the conference?"

I nodded.

"Anyway, I remember so vividly, when I was in college," Ellen continued. "I was a mess for sure, and yet coped and got good grades. I kept thinking that all that pain and grief with my father–that sexual-abuse stuff–must have something to do with my problems, with my headaches and stomach pains. I remember seeing the doctor at the university clinic. I even told him directly about the sexual abuse. I told him that I thought maybe some of my anxiety and my physical ailments were related to that past abuse stuff. I remember so plainly. He just said, "Look, here's some pills. You're a smart girl, just keep studying and you'll be okay. I remember how I felt silenced. Like I knew he didn't believe me or something. Anyway, it took three more attempts at various points in my life before I finally found a professional who listened."

"Ummm, that's sad, and when I think about it you were unusual in being able to directly tell the doctor about the abuse. And unusual in your insight into the fact that the abuse may be related to your physical problems. Although in the seventies no one talked about abuse the way we do now. But of course I realize in saying that how much I'm again just silencing you–saying that there were very good reasons why the doctor didn't hear you."

Again, we seemed to be in deep thought and were oblivious to the noise in the restaurant.

"I'm just thinking," I said. "I have this jumble in my brain. Women have stories of pain and symptoms so often connected to some way that they have been silenced. Doctors look for diagnosis, but that isn't often what it is about particularly for women. It so often has more to do with meaning–that is, symptoms are a way of trying to be heard. And yet how can a profession dominated by one gender hear what the other gender is saying? The doctor wants something concrete and black and white. The doctor wants to diagnose, fix, and label to feel secure. In other words, meaning for the doctor comes from feeling, in a sense, powerful about the ability to label and fix. And yet I wonder how much have women learned over centuries to express themselves in bodily terms or symptoms of some sort because that is the only way we will be heard. So without really realizing it, many women see physicians and express bodily symptoms because that is just the way of being in the world. And the doctor obviously doesn't want to know about experiences that can't be fixed by him. You know, the doctor at the university clinic didn't want to hear about your abuse. What could he do about it, and, even more scary, what if hearing about the way you were abused in any way reminded him of, you know, ways he may have been abusive? Does this make any sense? In other words, giving you pills and telling you to go away was really his way of protecting himself."

"Ummmm–I'm thinking–I have a glimpse of what you're saying," Ellen responded quickly. "I know I had no sense of being heard by those doctors and when I think about it the only way to even get their attention was with a body complaint. My body complaints were somehow legitimate and really what the doctor was comfortable with." Ellen paused for a moment and then continued. "After all though, aren't we all uncomfortable with this abuse stuff–you know, the sense that inside each of us is the ability to devalue someone? And really, that's what I experienced, the doctor's fear and discomfort about the issues. His need to reassure me that I was okay and that the pills would solve my body complaints were his way of controlling the situation. But unfortunately in the process I felt silenced and not heard, and the abuse issue of course didn't go away."

"Yes, I think I have a sense of what you experienced," I responded quickly. "It seems that often in the office I have this sense that women have learned to share information about their bodies with the doctor in a way that keeps the doctor comfortable and in control, so to speak." And then I felt confused and questioned. "But in that sense aren't doctors just part of the culture that has defined what women can do and say and what has value–you know, the sense that women are silenced because it is the male society that defines what has value, etcetera?"

"Yes, I agree," Ellen interjected quickly, "and of course doctors are part of the culture and there's no point in getting into a doctor-bashing agenda. But back to the communication stuff–that's what excites me, because that's what this is all about. How are women heard and how do they share what is important to them?"

I opened my mouth to respond but Ellen quickly motioned with her hand and continued. "That reminds me about a book I finished several months ago. About Alice James. She too was sick. Had the frail woman's body so prevalent in the upper-class women of the late 1800s. Anyway, I'm always looking for biographies about women–trying to find role models–trying to see how women have found answers. Come to think of it, her symptoms seemed to be the only way for her to express herself. Her brothers were those famous Jameses–you know, William the psychologist and Henry the writer.

Yes, women are the sick ones and maybe that's been the only way for so many women to be heard."

Now I felt excited. "Ellen, you make so much sense–and I must read that book. And I'm just sitting here thinking that I mentioned William James in one of my recent stories I've been writing, and I feel like suddenly something is coming together. I'm thinking clearly how one woman said to me just recently: 'When my head hurts I can't go out with him. The pain seems to be the only way I have to control my time with him. When I say, "Look, I'm in pain," he knows I won't budge on that. If I say "Look, I don't want to go out," he pesters me forever, so sometimes I just know I have to have pain.' At the same time I can hear so many other women saying: 'Look, I'm not stupid–this pain is in my body. What do you take me for?' And then I think, 'Of course we women are not stupid, but what if over the centuries we have just learned our social lessons well: how to be in the world and never threaten him; how to express ourselves in an indirect way because we just plain don't survive–in a physical or mental sense–if we are clear and direct. And what if the doctor needs to have labels and ways to fix us–that means we women need stories he is comfortable with because we have learned that the doctor is powerful and we musn't threaten him.' "

I realized I felt confused–even frightened. Ellen quickly sensed this and said, "This is scary stuff." We both sat there in thought. The waitress interrupted and took the plates. "Anything else today?" she asked.

"No, just the bill," I quickly responded and again looked at my watch.

"This is exciting," Ellen said. "I'll think about this business of body symptoms as a way to communicate."

"Uh, uh," I continued. "A way for women to be heard and in a strange sense the only way women often have of exerting control in their personal situations–I'll need to keep thinking about this."

We both moved out of our chairs quickly and then lingered at the table.

"Too bad, we have to go back to work and try to survive in the real world," Ellen said.

"But I guess that's where the challenge is," I said.

"And it's so good to just get some thoughts about all of this–being heard–stuff," Ellen said.

"You're right. Sometimes these thoughts swirl around my head and it's such a relief to get them out. Trying to put these ideas into words seems to be the only way to really look at the ideas. It's great sharing this stuff." I glanced at my watch.

"Yes, we have to get going," Ellen said, as we both collected ourselves and moved toward the door. "Look we must get together soon and talk more and I'll get you the book."

"Great, I look forward to reading it," I said.

As we walked out of the restaurant, I noticed for the first time that the place had been completely redecorated.

"Did you notice their new colors?"

She looked at me and then laughed.

"You do have your head in the clouds. I think they redid this place three years ago. Don't you get out much?"

"You're joking."

We quickly went our separate ways. As I walked down the sidewalk, I looked up and then I stopped abruptly. The sky–that incredible blue Alberta sky. I breathed deeply. The clouds were fluffy and white–spring clouds. I felt alive.

Chapter 14

Mary: The Dilemma

I always had a feeling, with my mother's talk and stories, of something swelling out behind. Like a cloud you couldn't see through, or get to the end of. There was a cloud, a poison, that had touched my mother's life. And when I grieved my mother, I became part of it. Then I would beat my head against my mother's stomach and breast, against her tall, firm front, demanding to be forgiven. My mother would tell me to ask God. But it wasn't God, it was my mother I had to get straight with.

–Alice Munro, *The Progress of Love*

MARY'S STORY

On Mary's first visit she quietly told me, "I just need more pills for my fibrositis." I sensed I could quickly write the prescription and that Mary and I would leave the room. I suspected she would just come back repeatedly and I would continue giving out pills. After all, she told me that this had been the problem for 15 years. Nothing had helped except the arthritis pills. They gave her some relief. She was switching doctors just because I was in a more convenient location. But she didn't see any reason to try anything new.

Mary sat there–waiting for the piece of paper. She looked older than 56, but it wasn't because of wrinkles. It had to do with a worn, exhausted, and resigned presence. Her clothes–drab, but neat and tidy. Her frame seemed to lack shape–nothing about her looked defined. Her greying hair hadn't seen a hairdresser for months.

I felt disconnected. I wasn't sure if I should even try to understand what the real Mary might be all about. I had to be honest. Fibrositis–more recently referred to as fibromyalgia–was a common problem, particularly with women. Generally, people with this difficulty frustrated me in some way. Fibromyalgia is characterized by ill-defined muscular aches and pains. In addition, there are a number of tender spots on the body that are extremely painful when pressed. Fatigue and depression complicate the diagnosis. Furthermore, the problem is tough to understand because there aren't any abnormal blood tests, and X rays or bone scans are normal. I felt tempted–don't bother trying to understand this disease. Just give her the pills and move to the next room. Other people waited with "real" problems I could fix.

But even if I couldn't understand fibromyalgia, I thought I had to struggle to know Mary in some fashion. I gave her more pills and suggested that she return for a complete checkup so I could know her better. She agreed. I felt certain she would return. I wished she had an easier label–like high blood pressure or even something tangible like diabetes or cancer.

Three Weeks Later

Mary looked the same on this visit–hair, clothes, and face unchanged. She could be one of those hundreds of women sitting at the bench in a factory–sewing, working, and not moving, but looking like you could push her over and no one would notice.

"So tell me about the pain," I said, as I began taking her history.

"I've had pain for 15 years," she responded carefully. "The mornings are bad. It's generally the worst in my neck and upper back. Some spots are so painful. Some mornings I can barely get out of bed. And sometimes I have pain in my shoulders and hips."

I nodded and said, "That sounds like fibromyalgia."

"It took the doctors a long time to diagnose me," she continued. "I had endless tests and X rays. But at least now I know what the problem is. As long as I don't push myself and take the pills I can at least cope."

"Sounds frustrating."

We agreed to continue the same approach for the pain problem. I wondered about physiotherapy but she had tried this a number of times. It didn't help much. I encouraged her to walk for exercise.

"Sometimes I do that," she said.

I continued asking questions.

"I've had four pregnancies," she said, "and they were all girls."

She told me they had left home and that all of them were healthy.

"I've had a hysterectomy and my gallbladder was taken out. If it wasn't for the pain I really would be quite healthy," she concluded.

I continued with the family history and reassured her I ask many questions about family health. Her parents had both died in their seventies. "My mother had arthritis," she said. "We were very close." Her father died of heart disease. She had two older sisters and they were both healthy.

"Any concern about alcoholism with either of your parents?" I questioned, as I reassured her that I ask everyone this question.

"Oh, no," she quickly responded. "My parents were wonderful. We were a close, Christian family. I never knew anything painful while growing up."

"Is your husband healthy?"

"Oh, yes, he's fine."

"Any concern with either you or your husband's use of alcohol?"

"Oh, no," she continued, "church is important to both of us and we never drink."

(At this point it can seem intrusive and inappropriate to ask about sexual or physical abuse, but experience had taught me to always raise this issue during complete checkups. People who are unable to deal with this issue can still choose to not reveal their problems.)

"Mary, this is a question I ask everyone," I said carefully. "Are you aware of any sexual or physical abuse to yourself or anyone else in the family?"

I watched her face as I talked and noticed her eyes immediately drop. Her hands–wringing.

Silence.

I waited.

Mary cleared her throat several times.

"Something hurts?" I questioned.

Mary nodded.

"Take your time, Mary," I said. "I can see it's painful."

And then she looked up.

"I really didn't want to talk about this, but since you've asked–yes–there has been sexual abuse. I'm not sure that it has anything to do with my health though–why are you asking anyway?"

"Mary, I ask this because I've come to understand that sometimes abuse affects us in ways we don't really understand."

"Maybe it won't hurt if I talk. Maybe it might help. Anyway, it's about my husband and daughter."

She stopped. She shifted in her chair. Her hands moved continuously. Her eyes stayed focused on the floor.

She sighed and looked up. "Anyway, it happened years ago and a while back my youngest daughter went to the police. I still have trouble believing all of this. They charged him. My daughter is so angry–and angry with me. Anyway, there was a court case. He's been ordered into therapy. You know–my daughter left home a few years ago. I don't know what she expected."

She stopped and looked up at me.

"That's it–I don't know how much it has to do with me–but I feel so torn."

"Are you talking to anyone?" I questioned, as I wondered how she could possibly handle this without support.

"Yes, I see the therapist also. Sometimes my husband and I go together and sometimes alone. The therapist is helping me. I don't know what it's doing to my husband. He's depressed and angry."

Her eyes dropped again.

"Sometimes I feel so confused. Andy's supposed to be the leader in the family. He never let me decide anything. I faithfully cared for the girls, did my church stuff–I know I've failed–but how could I have done it any different?"

And then she looked up. Her eyes filled with intensity and tears.

"I don't know, Mary," I said. "This sounds so painful."

Silence.

"You've shared so much with me Mary. I'm sure this must be tough."

She nodded.

I realized I couldn't possibly finish her physical exam that day. I talked to her more about her therapy and felt certain she was getting good support there. I questioned her about taking antidepressant medication, but she declined.

"I'm not sleeping, but I don't want any more pills," she said. Again she reminded me that she would be okay if she could just continue with the pills for her pain.

"It's just my body that hurts," she said.

I agreed again to continue her arthritis pills. I suggested she return in a week to finish her checkup. She agreed.

My mind wandered to Mary at the end of the day as I sat in my office staring at my charts. I felt stunned. I hadn't expected Mary to reveal anything abusive. I expected her to tell me everything in her family was okay. How little I really perceived about Mary. I daydreamed.

I pictured Mary in her living room, sitting on her sofa. Hands carefully folded. Ornaments placed on doilies. Immaculate carpet. No dust. And then she reached for the church papers and her Bible. She read. She understood. Her job. To be the perfect wife and mother. To submit to her husband and to God. It seemed easy. But she failed. She learned dependency so she could be the perfect wife. But how can dependency and invisibility make you a perfect mother? How could she protect her daughters?

I imagined her moving to her bedroom. I could see her looking critically at her body. Maybe it was just that her body didn't appeal to him. She noticed her sagging breasts, her rounded abdomen, and the dimples on her thighs. She wept. She crawled under her covers. She imagined a body more like her daughter's. Smooth silk skin, pretty compact breasts, and a flat stomach. Her body convulsed and I imagined her dead. After all, how could she respond to him after all those years of relentless criticism, intimidation, and persistent humiliation?

I jumped. Mary's pain overwhelmed me. I wondered what Mary would do, what would happen to her, how she would resolve her dilemma.

The Following Months

I saw Mary periodically. Her anguish remained incredible. Her physical pain escalated. She talked about her daughters. Her second daughter occasionally phoned her, but the other daughters refused to speak to her. I worried about her depression, but she continued to see the therapist and refused medication. I sensed that she rarely left her house except when she went to church and to the grocery store. She didn't know her neighbors and I gathered that she rarely talked to anyone. She talked less about her physical pain, although everything about her body movements screamed pain. Sometimes she mentioned her husband, although not often. And when she did I never really sensed anger. Rather there was sadness and an incredible sense of loss. Repeatedly she said, "How could this happen? I trusted him." And then she occasionally said, "What can I do?" I recognized her isolation. I encouraged every small step she took toward connection with other people.

One day she announced that her husband had finished therapy. "But nothing has changed," she said. "And he says it's my fault. I am too sick. I have too much pain. That I couldn't be a decent wife. I'm not sure though–was it all my fault?" she questioned.

When we had those kinds of conversations I concentrated on her strengths. I talked about all the tasks she had successfully completed. The way she had cared for her daughters. How she had accomplished a great deal in spite of her continual pain.

But sometimes I wondered. Would she be able to find the Mary that most certainly must exist? After years of continual invalidation with respect to everything about her, was it even reasonable to think that she could define herself in a new way?

One Year Later

Mary continued her counseling and I saw her only when she had physical concerns. I noticed small changes. On one occasion, when she came to see me because of a persisting sore throat, she talked about her friend from the church. She told me about their conversations. About how they struggled to understand how all of this had happened. I sensed that she made small steps in an attempt to address her dependency on her husband. She had no access to money and occasionally talked about getting a job. But on another occasion, I sensed the weight of her depression. A depression that appeared to never leave. Sometimes she mentioned her daughters. And always when she mentioned Heather–the youngest–

I sensed pain beyond comprehension. Occasionally she talked about leaving her husband. Inevitably she expressed remorse and a profound sense of failure. I continued to focus on her strengths and encouraged her self-expression. We no longer questioned the pain. Somehow the pain just made sense and finding ways to understand the pain while continuing to live seemed enough of a challenge for Mary.

One day she returned. This time her story had changed.

"I think I need physiotherapy for my neck," Mary volunteered. "And could you fill this form in?"

"Physio makes sense," I said, "but what's this form about?"

"I've left him." She looked at me–I sensed a weight had been lifted. "It's so hard," she continued. "I never dreamt I'd be on welfare, but if I could just have some time," and then she hesitated.

"Look, Mary," I said quickly. "This has to be tough for you. You've made a big step."

She nodded and then sighed, and her entire body slumped in the chair. But I sensed relief–yes, relief.

"I'm sure you need some time, Mary," I said, and then I realized she looked different–thinner, sharper, more defined.

She continued talking and seemed unconcerned about my presence: "I couldn't stand it any longer. He kept saying it was my fault. I'm sure some of it is–but it's dreadful–I just couldn't live with him anymore. But I'm so scared. I feel so alone. My apartment seems so empty. I'm 57. I've never lived alone. I wonder–can I survive?"

"Mary, you can survive."

"I can't believe it's come to this," she said. "Who am I? I have lost my family. No job. No skills. And the pain doesn't go away. The church says I should forgive him and that we must work it out. I just can't see it that way anymore."

"You are brave, Mary," I said.

We just sat there. We both seemed to need a moment to be quiet.

Silence.

I checked her neck and agreed physiotherapy was a good idea. I filled out the form. Diagnosis–depression and fibromyalgia. Expected time off–about three months.

Mary thought if she could just have three months to herself she'd be okay. She knew that the counseling helped and planned to continue this therapy. She had no idea what kind of job she could get but hoped she would figure something out. We talked about other support.

"Of course, I have my friend from the church," Mary said. "We still talk a lot. I think she understands how complicated this is for me. I really don't want to leave the church along with losing my family, but I think that's going to happen. It seems that I'm the problem–the crazy one, the sick one."

I listened to Mary and realized her strength inspired me.

"Come back in two weeks, Mary," I said, "and let me know how things are going."

I stayed in the examining room thinking about Mary.

Her pain no longer seemed mysterious. I wondered why there wasn't more pain. I felt angry. Why was it all Mary's fault? I wondered what all those years had been like for Mary. How could she possibly have been responsible for her husband's actions? What had it been like for her? The supportive and caring one. The one who couldn't decide, act, or set direction. The one who always followed. And maybe she hadn't always followed, but gave up trying to be heard. The one responsible for his unhappiness and anger–or so it seemed. How come her husband had stayed in the house, maintained his position in the church and community? Why did it seem that the daughters were more angry with their mother than with their father? How could this be? And Mary now had no financial security. She thought maybe she'd get something in the divorce but wasn't sure. She had paid a tremendous price for the social lessons she had learned so well–dependency, compliance. I felt exhausted thinking about the struggle it would be for Mary to find a new space in this world.

Two Years Later

The changes in Mary were gradual. She spoke with greater clarity. Her physical pain remained, but gradually lessened. She enrolled in classes at the college. On one occasion she talked about her fear.

"Now that I'm taking classes I sometimes feel I'm just motivated by fear. It seems I open my mouth just if I think it's necessary to please the teacher. I'm careful with my classmates. I don't do anything to disrupt anyone. I'm always afraid. Afraid I won't do it right. Afraid."

We continued to talk about the fear. It wasn't fear related to her sense of her physical self. It was always the fear of rejection. Sometimes she mentioned her past. Yes, her family had been caring and loving, but when she thought about it she sensed that their approval always depended on her being the perfect child, the right child, the quiet and compliant girl. She always felt like she might impose, might disrupt someone, might be a problem. But she began to heal. Slowly, she addressed the fears. I pointed out the steps she took. She continued to work hard with her therapist. Sometimes we talked about her spiritual journey. I knew Mary taught me and I told her so. Her anguish when the church dropped her name was tremendous. But she began to define her life in a new way. Her life took on new meaning–meaning where Mary had an existence.

She remained on welfare for a year. Eventually she found a job. It barely supported her but she gained confidence in herself and was relieved to be self-sufficient.

She worked in a women's clothing store as a clerk. Sometimes she described her fears at this job but occasionally she talked also about the fears she saw in other women who came looking for clothes. I sensed that for the first time in her life she was seeing the many ways women can be different, but also the many ways we may be similar. Sometimes she talked about the women who could never decide about the purchase–the women who she thought were paralyzed with fear.

"You know–you can just tell–they're worried if he'll like the blouse, if he'll approve. And it's not just the older women–some of the young women seem helpless. Sometimes I'm surprised how many women seem just like me."

And then we'd talk about women and fear and how we struggle to be heard.

One day she returned and announced, "I'm moving, so I'd like more arthritis pills and I just wanted to see you before I go."

"So what are you up to?"

"I'm moving to Kelowna. I have a sister out there and I've found a job that should be okay. I just decided I was ready for a change."

Mary looked different. I noticed the bracelets. She smiled and stretched. I realized she just looked alive. I hadn't understood how withdrawn–how dead–she really was those first few visits.

"Well, Mary," I said, "I'm going to miss seeing you. You've been a real inspiration."

We smiled.

Mary talked.

She told me about new experiences. Little things.

"He said I couldn't do anything right. I get my bills paid," and then she laughed. Hearing her laugh out loud made me feel alive.

"I just want a change of scenery," she said. "You know I've never actually lived somewhere when I made the decision about the place. We lived where he wanted to be. We went where he wanted to go. We ate breakfast when he was hungry."

"Ummmmm."

"Doesn't that sound crazy? I'm excited–sad–but excited. I can do it my way."

I gave her more arthritis pills. We stood up and Mary reached for the door.

"Mary, can we hug before you go?"

She smiled as we hugged. Mary opened the door and walked away.

Again I found myself paralyzed in the examining room. I just needed time to reflect about Mary.

Mary's independence, her strength, her growth, her autonomy–were now so apparent. Her pain seemed complex–just labeling her fibromyalgia didn't seem enough. Surely, she had been deprived of being a good mother because she had first been deprived of being a person. And now it seemed clear: her identity, her passion, her judgment, her feelings, her sexuality–buried in an avalanche of patriarchal garbage. Mary had struggled heroically. She had moved away and beyond the garbage.

Nine Years Later

I glanced at the chart before opening the door. Mary! I felt excited. She must be back. And then I noticed the new phone number and address. She had returned. I realized she had booked for a complete checkup.

I opened the door with anticipation.

Mary. She looked different. Her hair was white. The curls hung softly around her face. Her bracelets and earrings seemed too big, too bright for her and yet I loved them.

"Mary, it's so good to see you," I said.

"Yes, I'm glad to be back. I had a wonderful experience in Kelowna, but I wanted to come back."

She quickly filled me in. Her divorce had finally been settled and now that she was 65 she wanted to quit her job and retire. She had received some money with the divorce settlement, and with the government pension she could get by.

"I wanted to come back to Red Deer. Mostly it was to be closer to my daughters. We've started to talk more. And I realized I missed a few old friends. Being in Kelowna really worked, but I'm glad to be back. I guess this is sort of home to me and I realize that now."

"It's wonderful to see you, Mary, and you look great."

She quickly talked about her youngest daughter.

"Heather and I are talking now," she said. "Heather lives in Edmonton. We talk on the phone and get together. It's such a good feeling for me. Heather's marriage fell apart three years ago and now she's getting counseling. Finally we can talk about the sexual abuse."

"Mary, I'm glad you and Heather are talking."

"Some of it still hurts so much–Heather's counselor says I must have known everything. But it's strange, you know–I really didn't know what was going on."

We both were quiet.

"Ummmmm," I murmured, and then realized I was sort of thinking and talking out loud and not sure what I was really saying.

"But Mary, maybe you were just really busy–keeping the house clean and the girls in ironed clothes, keeping his meals cooked just right, keeping out of trouble yourself. Maybe–maybe–you know Mary–I don't know, sometimes to be honest, I just think we all have bought this notion, this idea that our mothers can be everything for us. Where did this idea come from? I think it's a myth–a myth that this culture perpetuates, the myth of the all-wonderful, all-compassionate and caring mother. How can any of us fill that role? And how could you fill that role when you didn't have any power, any say in how things were decided?"

I stopped.

Mary looked squarely at me.

"Those are the best words I've ever heard," she said.

I blinked.

"I did my best–I know that," she said. "I just hope that someday Heather will understand that."

We sat there. Silent. Quiet. And more quiet.

"Oh, Mary," I said, needing finally to break the moment. "How you've grown!"

Silence.

"Yes–I have. I exist. I have glimpses of peace."

And then we got on with the checkup.

Mary still took arthritis pills, but not all the time. Physically she was healthier than I had ever seen her. I ordered the mammogram, ordered the blood tests–and Mary agreed–everything was going well so she'd just come in for the occasional checkup.

This time when Mary left, I sat in my office. I couldn't see another patient until I felt what I needed to feel. I sat there.

I thought about Mary, her daughter. About all daughters. All mothers. Something hurt so much. We blame. We want our mothers to be everything. They never can. We are angry with them. They always fail us. And then finally we grow up. Finally we can see. It isn't our mothers who have failed. It's this crazy system. This myth. The myth that mothers are powerful. But their power always has strings attached.

That day I could see–my own mother–her poison–my poison–and where my daughter too would be poisoned. That day I finally glimpsed something. For Mary to heal, for me to heal, for my mother to heal, for my daughter to heal, for women to heal, we needed a glimpse of Mary and Heather–reaching out, understanding each other, writing new rules, Mary's hand reaching her mother, and then Mary's hand reaching Heather, and then Heather reaching her daughter, and on and on and on.

PART III.
THE HEALING JOURNEY

The best and most beautiful things in the world cannot be seen or even touched. They must be felt with the heart.

–Helen Keller, *The Story of My Life*

Chapter 15

Healing and Chronic Pain: Practical Ideas

> Anna wasn't ready for how painful it was to watch this–painful as a bird beating against the unyielding transparency of glass. She wanted to be the child dancing beside the woman, holding her hands through the bars. She wanted to take an axe and chop right through them, set the caged dancer free.
>
> –Janice Kulyk Keefer, *Rest Harrow*

THE CHRONIC PAIN DILEMMA

In the story in Chapter 1 Sharon comes to my office with an immediate agenda. Most of the initial visit is about Sharon and her general frustration with doctors because her pain problem has not been fixed. This is a common scenario in my office.

I hear comments such as:

> I just haven't been satisfied with doctors. They've given me these pills. They've done X rays and took blood tests. They say there's nothing wrong. The pills bother my stomach and besides they say I'll just have to live with the pain. I'm only 54 and I'm not ready for that. I know this isn't in my head.

Or:

> I've gone to a walk-in clinic. They never seem to have time to listen to me. They've sent me to three specialists but they just

> seem to have their own list of questions and when they're satisfied I'm not diseased I'm out of there. No one seems to want to listen to me.

If you have pain and are feeling stuck, as Sharon was, it is likely you have a chronic pain problem. As I mentioned in a previous chapter, doctors and patients have minimal difficulty with acute pain problems. If you've broken your leg, sprained your ankle, developed appendicitis, or are in the midst of a gallbladder or heart attack, quite likely you can find doctors who listen and act quickly.

But now, the story is different. It's been seven months since the car accident and you still have neck pain. It's been a year with stomach pain and no one can find the problem or you have headaches every week and this has been an issue for five years. You and your doctors are frustrated and confused.

How Can You Proceed in a Different Fashion?

As you recall in Sharon's story, on the first visit we discussed the need for a different approach and the need for both of us to work together. I believe anyone with a chronic pain problem must struggle with their own readiness to become actively involved with their pain problem. There are rarely simple "cures" to chronic pain problems. The willingness to become involved will likely occur over time. As you gain more confidence in a different approach, you will be less reliant on others to magically solve your problems. And you need a doctor who is willing to work with you from that perspective.

What Kind of Doctor Do You Need?

You need a doctor who specializes in primary care and one who understands your need for continuity of care. You want someone who is willing to take a good history and listen to you. You and your doctor will both need to be willing to look beyond the magic of the fantasy cure. You need a doctor who is willing to see you as the expert for your own health, and you in turn need to understand that you must get involved and be that expert. "So what does that mean," you ask, "and how do I find this doctor?"

In Canada, you likely will have minimal difficulty locating physicians who call themselves family or general practitioners. In the United States, there may be more difficulty, but if you know that's what you're looking for, you probably will be able to locate a family physician or someone with training in primary care.

If you already have a primary-care physician, you might ask yourself a few questions. Have you been able to talk about what you want to talk about? Have you had a complete checkup recently, and are there any problems in trying to book this? Can you talk to your doctor about concerns with respect to how your problems are addressed? Are you willing to really work on getting involved with your health? In addition, ask yourself: What does your doctor know about you? Does he/she know whom you live with, what your job is, whether you have financial concerns, or whether you're worried about your kids or your partner? Family physicians should want to know those kinds of things. If you've seen your doctor for a while and he or she knows little about you, and aren't asking or listening if you do try to talk about this stuff, you may need to try a new doctor. But remember, if you are switching often, you are not giving yourself or your doctor a chance to really address the concerns.

If you realize that you go to one specialist for your pap smear and another for your high blood pressure and then to the walk-in center for your sprained ankle and now can't find someone who is willing to talk about your headaches, find a family physician. The generalist physician is trained to think about your whole body and is most able to think about your need for continuity of care.

If you can't remember ever seeing a doctor where you really told your whole story of chronic pain and had a checkup then this is where you start. Call the doctor's office and book for a complete checkup.

The complete checkup starts first with you giving the doctor your medical story. This is an opportunity for you to tell your pain story and to give your doctor a sense about your life. The doctor will check your body, and you and the doctor will talk about diagnostic tests. From this information, you and the doctor can begin to formulate an understanding of the chronic pain problem and proceed with a plan for managing the pain.

That sounds straightforward, but often is very complex. Let's look at each part of this process.

Telling the Doctor Your Story

Your doctor has an agenda–what he/she thinks needs to be known about you. But you have a list–what you think he/she needs to know about you and the pain. I'll help you write your list. It's useful to go to the doctor prepared. Doctors are busy. They have bad days. They may be preoccupied with other concerns when you get there. If you've written things down, it's easier for you and them.

1. The Chronic Pain Story

Tell this story from beginning to end–give dates, investigations, doctors you've seen, etc. Give information about the present pain story.

For example:

> The headaches started eight years ago. They seemed to come from nowhere. At first they weren't too bad and I just took Tylenol. After three years they got worse. I saw a specialist. He said they were tension headaches. I tried some kind of pills then–I took them every day–but they didn't help. In the last year they've become worse. Now I have daily headaches. The pain always starts in the back of my neck and works up to the top of my head, etc.

Your doctor should ask you specific questions. Talk about the present pain problem until you feel as if you've explained the story.

2. Your Past Health Problems

Your doctor needs to know what surgeries you've had and about major medical problems. Again, it's useful to prepare a list. For example: 1947 my appendix out, 1963 hysterectomy, 1975 a bad pneumonia, etc.

3. Your Family History

Your doctor will likely need help with this. Some of this information your doctor may not want to hear, but persist. It's my experience that when I find out more about peoples' lives, I come to appreciate their perspective easier.

Start with your parents. Give a quick summary. Are they healthy, or if they've died, do you know what from? Remember, if one or both of your parents had an alcohol or drug problem, your doctor can benefit from knowing this. If your parents' health is a concern for you now, talk about it. If you're the major support system for a parent, mention that. Give a summary of any major health concerns for your siblings.

Think about the overall picture while you were growing up. If your parents divorced when you were five and then you lived with your mother and eventually a stepfather, mention this. If you lived in three foster families, that's important. If you experienced abuse, ask yourself if you're ready to tell anyone about this. Doctors in the past haven't been particularly trained to ask about abuse, although more doctors in training now are getting education about abuse as a health issue. Your doctor will know, however, where you can go if you want to talk to someone about your experience. Think about this. If a history of abuse is part of your story and you don't want to talk to your doctor, you might think about finding a mental health counselor or other therapist. If you've been in therapy and are experiencing a healing journey, you can tell your doctor.

If your husband/partner has health problems, or if you have relationship issues, it is important to mention this. If your partner abuses you–emotionally, physically, or sexually–this is important to discuss. Ask yourself about your safety and discuss this if you are concerned. If you're in a lesbian relationship, you may want to tell your doctor that as well.

Give a quick summary of any health concerns or behavioral issues with children.

4. Your Social History

Give a quick summary of your job. If you're new to Canada or the United States, give your doctor a summary of where you're from and something about how you came to move to a new country. If your culture is different from your doctor's, don't hesitate to educate him/her. If financial worries are an issue or you lack financial independence, talk about that.

5. Other Things

Your doctor needs to know if you smoke, if you drink alcohol or take drugs, whether you have allergies, or if you exercise. Be fair. Give an accurate picture. Otherwise, you're wasting your time and the doctor's.

Once you've finished giving the information you think is important and the doctor has obtained information he/she thinks is relevant, the next step is the physical examination.

Your Body–The Physical Examination

The physical examination should include a focus on the part of the body where you experience the pain, but also must include an assessment of the entire body. Is your blood pressure normal? What about those spots on your skin or that lump on your leg? This is your chance to point out any physical concern that you may have. This is also your opportunity to talk about preventive health procedures, such as a mammogram and pap test, and for you to have these tests done. Talk about how often to be checked. You should have a sense that your body has been checked. If you have any concerns about what your doctor is doing, you should ask him/her to explain.

Investigation of the Pain Problem

Once the doctor has your story and has completed the physical examination, you are ready to discuss further investigation of the pain problem. Your doctor should be able to give you a clear picture of what he/she understands up to this point from the history and physical examination. Then, you will need to discuss what diagnostic tests are needed or what referrals to specialists would be appropriate. This is where you and the doctor need to struggle to find balance. No investigation may mean missing problems where the pain is directly related to something in the body that can be fixed or treated in a straightforward fashion, while continual focus on yet one more test, hoping to find the elusive fix, may create frustration and even greater problems. Finding this balance will be an ongoing concern for you and the doctor. For most chronic pain problems, once the history, physical examination, and tests have been completed, you will either have a sense that the pain is related to a chronic problem that doctors have an understanding of but can't cure–such as cancer or rheumatoid arthritis–or you will be left with the sense that your pain problem is not related to any disease in the body that has a clear pathological identity–as is the case with irritable bowel syndrome, fibromyalgia, or tension headaches. This is where it becomes difficult. I regularly struggle with patients with the notion that just because the X ray is normal or the blood tests are alright doesn't mean that I think the pain is just in their head. You and the doctor need to continue talking until there is a sense of understanding the situation.

Understanding and Living with Chronic Pain

I find it useful to schedule periodic visits to monitor the pain problem. If the story changes or the pain escalates, the situation can be reassessed. For most pain problems, it is useful to aim for control of the problem, rather than expecting complete resolution of the pain problem.

What else can women do about the pain?

Over the years, I have listened to many women, and often I'm struck with the diversity of approaches that women take to deal with their pain. I'll summarize some of these ideas.

If you're stuck with chronic pain inevitably you will need to get brave and try something new! Ask yourself how you care for your body. Yes, you will need to address those health habits. If you're obsessed with diet and exercise–give yourself a break. If you don't exercise at all, I suggest you start walking or doing something even if the pain seems to worsen initially. If you smoke, you're not doing yourself a favor. If you've been seeing a physiotherapist for your painful back or neck and it's not helping, then you might try a massage therapist, for example. The point is that when you're stuck with the pain and there is no change, then make a change. I am becoming convinced that the main issue is the person having a sense of direction that comes from within. A sense that they are no longer counting on the magic out there, but are beginning to find the magic within themselves. That doesn't necessarily mean that the pain goes away, but often it means that women are able to find new perspectives that allow them to live more productive lives in spite of their pain.

Look at whom you talk with and spend time with. Make changes. Look at the pattern of support in your family. Do you support everyone? Then you might want to back off. Get help in figuring this out if you need to. Or, if everyone supports you, then see a therapist and figure out how to become more self-sufficient. Look at your support outside the family and make changes if that seems appropriate. For some women this has meant joining a church group, for instance, or joining a twelve-step program. Paradoxically, for other women it has meant leaving their groups! What about your friends? Are you everyone's support person, or do your friends give you support?

Often I see the chronic pain story somehow tied to the way women have been silenced and have learned patterns of behavior to survive abuse issues. For that reason, it may be helpful to seek counseling. However, you will need to talk to someone who has a sense that you can heal. Again, I have noticed how women who are seeing therapists may magically improve physically when they either switch therapists or stop therapy. Healing is about learning to trust your inner knowledge and becoming who you really are. Find a therapist with that vision.

Take a sensible approach with your doctor around the pain medication scenario. There's no point in denying yourself medication that can be helpful and can give you a more productive life. Conversely, don't become addicted to narcotics and tranquilizers and create a new problem. If you use alcohol to numb your pain, see an addiction counselor. Always try to find the balance.

The Continuation of the Pain Story

This is where it becomes important to have a primary-care physician who understands the chronic pain story. This business of pain so often mirrors the processes of our lives. I see people getting better and people getting worse, often without a clear understanding of what's happening. Sometimes we need to investigate vigorously and other times we need to wait. You and your doctor need to work together. Continuity of care is extremely important. Sometimes what you may need is the sense of curing and at other times the caring factor will be more important.

Depression can often be a big part of the pain story. Depression can respond to medication, but, again, the issues are complex. Sometimes I am struck by the sense of the mystery of this pain business. Someone will come back to see me and the heaviness of her pain seems to have lifted. Often in these situations, people will be able to articulate clearly how they believe they have begun to heal. At other times, there will be an understanding of willingness to simply continue living with greater acceptance of physical pain.

Inevitably, however, healing from chronic pain is tied to greater self-knowledge and expression. It is the mystery of this healing process that I explore in the next section.

Chapter 16

Healing and Chronic Pain: Reflective Ideas

I hung on the wall the work I had been doing for several months. Then I sat down and looked at it. I could see how each painting or drawing had been done according to one teacher or another, and I said to myself, "I have things in my head that are not like what anyone has taught me–shapes and ideas so near to me–so natural to my way of being and thinking that it hasn't occurred to me to put them down." I decided to start anew–to strip away what I had been taught–to accept as true my own thinking.

–Georgia O'Keeffe, *Georgia O'Keeffe*

THE MYSTERY–WHAT STARTS THE HEALING JOURNEY?

Sometimes, when thinking about Sharon and other women I see in my practice, I sense mystery. What gets someone started on a healing journey? It's a mystery how some women begin to heal and start their journeys. It's also equally mysterious how women struggle in pain and anguish for so long before taking different steps. Healing from chronic pain is complex. Of course, it's about so much more than just pain in our bodies. Inevitably healing is a personal experience.

When I saw Sharon on that first visit and suggested we would need to work in a different way, I had no idea whether she would return. Healing from chronic pain requires willingness to become actively involved in the process. That means taking responsibility. It means there is no magic pill. I've come to understand that it is not my job to know when someone is willing to work in a different way. My part is to have a vision that the person can take her own steps and that she will take these steps when she is able.

In thinking about how I see women begin to take a different approach with their chronic pain problems, I'm struck by two opposing scenarios. There are stories much like Sharon's, where it seems that in a rather dramatic fashion a big change occurs. Something really clicks and the person says–yes, it's up to me.

But more often the healing journey begins in a less dramatic fashion. Often there is no clear sense of the beginning. Barbara is a woman I often think about when contemplating the complexity of the beginnings of healing stories.

I've worked with Barbara for several years. Barbara is 28, and her story is one of drama and contrasts. She had a chaotic past–father who abandoned her, mother who remarried and created more children, and a new father who sexually abused her. Barbara never belonged in the new family. Barbara grew up confused and alone. Now Barbara has a good job, but creates endless problems for herself with her inconsistent work habits. She has illness. Allergies. Her eczema, hay fever, and asthma are difficult to control. Her headaches persist. And then the labels–borderline personality disorder, major depressive disorder, panic disorder. Her entire body and psyche seemed enveloped in pain and confusion.

When Barbara first came to see me a few years ago, I can't say that I wanted her as a patient. She was difficult. I struggled to be consistent with managing the problems. I set firm guidelines about appointments, about her medication, about seeing her therapist. And sometimes she complied and sometimes she didn't. Over the course of a few years she was in and out of the hospital. She spent time on the psychiatric ward for her suicide attempts and on the medical ward for her asthma that was out of control because she didn't take her medication and persisted in smoking.

I watched. I cared. I understood that Barbara, with her flamboyant clothes and face bursting either with tears or laughter, was on her own journey. One day Barbara came for renewal of her medication and said, "It's up to me, isn't it?"

"Ummmm, yes," I said.

And then she proceeded to talk about her weekend and her thoughts about suicide, about the headaches, about the depression, about the asthma.

"I can't even do myself in," she said. "I'm that bad."

"Oh, I suppose that's one way of looking at things," I said. "But there's another interpretation."

"Like what?"

"Well, the way I see things, Barbara, I sometimes imagine that you walk along a cliff. Periodically, you slide over the edge and reach out just in time–you catch therapists' hands, your friends' hands, or sometimes you're completely on your own and grab for safety just in time. In the midst of this you've also walked away from the cliff. You've tried every conceivable approach–the group therapy situation, the cognitive therapy, the behavioral approach. But, I think you're beginning to see. It's really up to you. So, it's not that you're all bad and can't even do yourself in–as you say–but rather that you're working hard, trying to get away from the cliff. Others can lend you a hand, but ultimately it is up to you. That's the way I see it. You have to walk away from the cliff. No one can make your feet take those steps."

She interrupted quickly.

"You're right, because I know if I really wanted to do myself in–jump off the cliff as you say–there is nothing ultimately that you as my doctor or any of my therapists can do that will stop me."

My mouth felt dry.

"You're right, Barbara. So, it's up to you."

We sat silently.

And then I continued.

"But if you turn just a bit, Barbara, and walk away from the cliff, there are other possibilities for you. There is a big field out there–brush in the field, but some flowers. You could begin to find a few flowers."

Again we sat in silence.

And then Barbara talked more about her job and her direction in her life. Over the next few months, I gradually sensed that Barbara indeed moved in a new direction.

I continue to see Barbara. That day represented a slight shift. I no longer wonder about the mystery of the beginnings of healing journeys. I accept that the beginnings happen. I understand that to heal from chronic pain and the depression that inevitably is part of the story requires willingness to begin to say: "Yes, it's up to me." It means willingness to say: "Okay, I understand I experienced some crummy stuff while growing up but I won't blame my parents forever. I'll get with it." It may mean: "Yes, my husband feels like an incredible stumbling block, but I'll either start to figure out how to leave or I'll figure out how to achieve my own goals while we're under the same roof." It means: "I'll begin to define who I am. I will set limits. I will be realistic about the dangers in my life. I will move from my helpless, hopeless position and begin to be who I am." It means: "I will stop looking for the magic cure for the pain and begin to find new approaches." It means: "I have a sense of the ways women are squished in this culture but even that won't stop me. I will stop throwing bricks. I will begin to lay bricks in a new fashion and create my own space. I will be who I am."

THE MYSTERY OF BODY PAIN– DO I NEED TO LEARN TO HEAR MY BODY?

Sometimes I'm struck by the paradox of women in pain. On the one hand, the pain is so obvious. They hurt. Their necks and back hurt. Their stomachs ache. They have pelvic pain. Their heads hurt. Their physical pain is so evident–evident on their faces–evident in their descriptions. Women in pain are obvious in medical clinics. They fill up the waiting rooms. They line up in hospitals for surgery. And yet so often they feel that no one believes them or can help them. Their tests are normal. It's so simple–fix the pain.

On the other hand, maybe the pain isn't going away because it's not so simple. Maybe it's not so obvious what the problem is. Maybe the pain is symbolic of much more than body pathology. But maybe none of us–doctors or patients–really want to struggle with difficult stuff. We want it to be simple. Simple straightforward tests and simple solutions. Patients and doctors don't want to get into the tough stuff. Don't ask me about the meaning in my life, whether I'm the doctor or the patient. Let me keep it superficial and simple. Just let me give you pills and tests, and you keep taking your pills–let's none of us rock the boat.

Because the flip side of the simple solution is inevitably complex. It means that women will have to ask tough questions. It means everyone will have to seek complex solutions.

It means that women will have to listen to their bodies, in the way Sharon learned to hear her body. It means we will have to stop trying to control our bodies and instead get reacquainted with them and begin to listen to their messages. And who wants to embark on this journey when the culture pushes you on the simple pathway? I'm beginning to see that it means understanding that in this culture all women experience abuse in some sense–it is the sense of the feminine that is so abused, denied, and silenced. It is the sense that the part of you that is intuitive, that feels emotion, that is connected and opposite to the rational and self-sufficient masculine sense, that is so silenced. Somehow in this process of silencing of the feminine voice we see women in pain–women dissociated from the meaning of the pain in their bodies–women no longer connected to their own bodies.

In the story in Chapter 1, Sharon said, "I still have pain, but I'm not so afraid now. When my neck starts to hurt sometimes I can even see that I've been working too hard or not getting enough rest or something. I think my body does give me some signals that are meant to help me. I'm really trying to pay attention to my body now. I'm sure this sounds crazy."

And I said, "Not at all, Sharon."

What seems so simple is really so complex. It was no easy task for Sharon to reach the point where she verbalized her pain story in those words.

I'm reminded of Kathy when thinking about body messages and their meaning. Kathy, who was in her fifties and struggling in a difficult marriage, talked about her pain in this way.

"Sometimes, I'm sure my neck bothers me more when I don't want to go out with him. He just won't take no for an answer, but if I say my neck pain is worse, then I don't have to go."

Kathy had talked on many occasions about her past and present dilemma. Growing up she remembers how pain played a big part in her life. It seems that she could never talk about what really bothered her. If she felt worried or concerned about anything and tried to express this, inevitably she heard: "Don't think like that," or "Those feelings about your sister are bad," or "What will Aunt Jane think?" or "What will the church think," or "What would your teacher say?" Inevitably it seemed as Kathy put it: "That the only way to express any emotional content was in the form of words about body pain."

And so, in time, Kathy became less and less aware of what her feelings really were. She tuned into her body responses with minimal awareness of the connection to her emotional life. So when she had a bad experience in school, for example, she didn't go home and talk about it. She only knew that her stomach hurt and that's what she talked about. And who knows what really happens to our bodies over time, when we keep experiencing stress but repeatedly block awareness of the emotional response?

To begin to listen to the pain in our bodies and to begin to understand that the pain messages are complex–are related to our emotional selves, are related to what may be buried, are related to physical changes that occurred over time–is no simple task. To begin to communicate with our partners and other people in a direct fashion when they may not want to hear our truth requires a giant step. For Kathy to clearly state, "No, I will not go out with you tonight," and then to solidly be clear about her intentions and be able to stand clear from his inevitable objection is tough. No wonder women sometimes unconsciously remain with the pain story–it is serving a useful purpose.

But the challenge–whether the individual woman in pain is willing to begin to connect with her body–is to begin to see the complexity, to begin her own healing journey. The challenge is to be part of new voices in a culture that has lost the voice of the feminine. The challenge is to begin to speak your own truth.

THE MYSTERY–IS THE FLIP SIDE OF PAIN REALLY JOY?

In the story in Chapter 1, I comment at the end: "She continued to have pain but it no longer dominated her life. . . . She continued to find new ways to understand and be Sharon."

Repeatedly, I see women move into that phase of their healing process–I call it joy. Often, their bodies still hurt. They may still have fibromyalgia, irritable bowel syndrome, or may still have pain from their cancer or rheumatoid arthritis. These women have taught me and inspire me. Inevitably their healing is about connecting with something within themselves and beginning to direct their lives from a new perspective. It means that they have moved out of the blaming phase and found their own path.

This is the part of the story with no formula. No easy steps for me to give patients and no easy tests to tell other doctors to give.

I'm reminded of Marilyn. Marilyn had been in my practice for several years. I watched her heal and find joy. She had the usual stuff–abuse, parental neglect, marriage to an alcohol-dependent man. Her diagnosis was fibromyalgia, and her pain had been complicated by an injury that left her with a painful ankle. Over the years, I watched her struggle and watched her find joy and peace. It didn't happen overnight. It didn't happen with fireworks or balloons. It happened because Marilyn made it happen.

She went to groups, she worked with physiotherapists, she created her own spiritual path. Her pain has not disappeared, but her pain is no longer the focus of her life. Recently, she talked about her new involvement with a volunteer organization. As she talked, I noticed the smile, the way her hands relaxed on her lap, the way Marilyn–the authentic real Marilyn–shone in my office. And I knew–joy isn't found in pill bottles. But pain and joy do go hand in hand. That's what is difficult for all of us.

THE MYSTERY OF PAIN AND WOMEN'S SPIRITUAL JOURNEY

A few years ago, I probably would not have even noticed Marilyn's joy or thought about her and the ways she seemed real in the office. Ideas about pain, joy, and spirituality didn't sound much like anything to do with diagnosing and treating chronic pain problems. But somewhere back there I began to see, and Elise played her role in beginning to open my eyes.

The story begins with Elise and Muriel. Both were women in their seventies. Both of them were diagnosed with lung cancer. Both of them received the usual care from their cancer specialists, and eventually both were admitted to the hospital when they could no longer cope with their pain and palliative care was needed. I was their doctor.

By the time of their admissions I had known both women for several years, although neither had been in my practice for a long time and I did not have the connection with either of them that I often share with women I've known for a decade. Daily, I made rounds in the hospital (that means you go to the wards, talk to the patients, talk to the nurses, write new orders, etc.) and visited Muriel and Elise. Both women experienced major pain and were on high doses of morphine. Their cancers had spread to their bones and this accounted for the escalating pain.

In time, I gradually noticed that a pattern developed in my rounds. I would first go the postpartum ward and then head up to the medical wards. I always went to Unit 37 first and saw Muriel. Then, I'd head over to Unit 38 and visit Elise. If I had other places to go, I'd inevitably arrange things to make my visit to Elise the last visit before going to my office. Occasionally, I wouldn't get everything finished and would head back to the hospital at noon to see Elise.

I understood that my visit to Unit 37 seemed difficult. Muriel's questions, complaints, agitation, and general unhappiness challenged me. Inevitably, she wondered when she would go home. Inevitably, she talked about the things she still wanted to do. I understood that hope was important, but I always felt somehow disjointed when I saw Muriel. And then the family issues were complex–phone calls from family members, consultations with family members in the hospital. Oh, I understood the family dynamics. I understood that Muriel had played the strong mother role and that her grown children continued to rebel. I involved the social worker, arranged visits home when she was able, and struggled to stay focused on Muriel's needs.

Sometimes I sat back and thought about the richness of her life. Muriel had five grown children who were all married. She had many grandchildren. Her husband had died, but left her financially secure. She played an active role in her church and in her community. It made sense to me that she struggled with her diminishing role, with her increasing pain, and with her impending death.

And so I would leave Unit 37 and head over to Unit 38. I would still be thinking about Muriel. Wondering if there was anything else I could do to help her. Wondering if Muriel would stop talking about what she planned to do when she left the hospital. Wondering if the intense pain would ever subside. With Muriel I realized we were somehow always in the tomorrow phase. Somehow, we never quite seemed to be in the today phase.

It seemed that making my visit to Unit 38 the last visit on my rounds happened gradually. I wasn't really aware of the process. I just noticed after both had been in the hospital for about a month that I always ended on Unit 38.

Elise seemed to lack the drama of Muriel. There were fewer family issues by the very fact that she had only one child and one grandchild. Her daughter lived in a different province, so of course she could not visit daily. Elise had friends. They visited. I knew Elise suffered greatly from her pain as well, but I realized we did not talk a lot about the pain.

One day while driving to the office it dawned on me: "Can't you see? When you visit Elise you feel better; you feel blessed." I wiped the tears from my eyes that day while in my car as I drove from the hospital. I thought, "Yes, that's it. When I spend time with Elise I feel calm, I feel settled, I feel whole. But how can this be?" I wondered. "She has so much pain and she's dying. This pain is so connected to her body–so easy to see that the pain is from her bones."

And so I gradually listened more to Elise.

Sometimes she joked. Sometimes her bluntness caught me off guard. It wasn't that Elise was peaches and cream, I realized. But I began to see that with Elise everything seemed real–seemed today–seemed authentic and now.

"I don't like that bird seed," she said one day, referring to the laxative. "Can't you do better than that?"

I laughed. "I'm sure we can try something else."

It was simple. She didn't expect miracles, but she wanted to be heard.

One day I think I must have said, "Tell me, Elise–what is your secret?"

She looked perplexed. "What are you talking about?"

"Oh, you seem content," I said.

"Life isn't that complicated, you know. When I got sick two years ago, I had to move out of my house to an apartment. I moved closer to the store and the church. I could walk for my groceries and walk to the church. I never really went to church much, but I've always prayed. I needed time for myself."

And we'd talk more.

One day she said, "Look, this is for my granddaughter."

"What is that?"

"I'm writing a letter to her–something she will be able to read when she's older. There are things I want to share with her."

"That's wonderful."

That day I vividly recall leaving the hospital in my car. I stopped on the street next to the hospital where tall old poplars line the street beside small old houses. I felt my own solitude. It seemed clear. Elise lived in the present. Elise wasn't waiting for tomorrow. Elise wasn't waiting to please someone else, or to expecting her doctors to fix her. Elise listened to something within herself. Her pain never went away, but somehow she transcended the pain. Truly, Elise connected with me from her own strong inner sense of herself. That's what attracted me to her–that's why I felt blessed.

Elise and Muriel died within one week of each other. I missed them.

The pain story is complex. And yet, when women begin to connect with that strong center within themselves, I'm amazed at the journeys I see them embark on. Their paths are all unique. Their stories of abuse and of being silenced are as varied as the rituals they create in healing. But, inevitably, healing from chronic pain is about finding and trusting that inner wisdom within yourself.

Chapter 17

The Old Concrete Culvert

> She wanted to be certain. To know. To know not, as she thought, philosophy, but something more important. The truth. The truth for her. Not always to be torn, to wonder if . . .
>
> –Marian Engel, *The Glassy Sea*

I found the path. The path started at the barn, crossed a small stream, and curved over the knoll of the hill before descending toward the coulee. The coulee was a small valley just south of the farm where I grew up. At the bottom of the coulee there was a small dirt dam that created a watering hole for the cows. You could cross over the dam to the south side of the coulee or stay on the north side.

It had been years since I walked this path–a path the cows always followed to the pasture, and a path I always followed to find the cows and bring them home at night. On that day I just wanted to find the path and walk.

I remembered one year, in the spring, how the dam burst from the runoff, and the road at the bottom of the hill was washed out. After that they put in a big culvert. The new shiny culvert and higher, bigger road never seemed quite like they belonged. I loved the old concrete culvert. It seemed to fit, even if it couldn't do the job.

On that day, I walked on the north side of the coulee. The trail followed close to the water, sometimes in thick brush and in other places wide open space. I remembered that it was always a guess which side of the coulee to look for the cows first, and always annoyance when you saw them directly across from you and that meant walking all the way back to the dam to get to the other side. The hills on both sides of the coulee had wonderful pasture. Of course, that's why the cows were kept there. But it had been years since there were cows in this pasture. And so trees had grown over the path–willows touched me from both sides.

I walked along, staring at my feet–watching where I placed my running shoes. Oops–I stepped over a dried-out cow pie and burst into laughter. That's why I'm watching my feet. I had forgotten.

I walked further. Took in the scenery. The blue sky. A wonderful fall day. The orange leaves on the poplar trees clinging to the branches. I got glimpses of the wheat field at the top of the hill. Harvest time. I had come back once more to the family farm to see the combines–all five of them–picking up the swath and miraculously pouring wheat into the big trucks.

I felt alone. I felt the stillness. I felt the solitude. I relaxed.

But just when I felt certain I could have an easy, comfortable walk, the committee in that secret part of my head started in. You know–there is that public part of yourself that everyone sees, there is the private part of yourself that husbands, close friends, or lovers see, and then the secret part of yourself that even you are not always aware of and are often confused by.

I often envision the secret part of myself to be a committee. The members of the committee meet sporadically and often struggle for my attention when I least want to hear them.

And so, on that day, I realized I had gradually fallen into thoughts about the women who come to my office. I had been thinking about Sharon–from the story in Chapter 1–thinking how real my experience with her had felt. Thinking about other women who have experiences where I think: "Wow, such clarity. She's moved beyond her confused and painful state into something so powerful." Experiences where it seemed so clear that healing from chronic pain, depression, anxiety, eating disorders, and so much more of what I see, is about becoming who you are. And yet my own sense of clarity wasn't there.

The committee was at it again. The rational voice on the committee spoke loud and clear. There was no drama to his voice. Just solid, rigid, unmoving dialogue.

"Look–wake up," the rational voice continued. "You're a doctor–claim to be sort of a scientist. You know better than to believe what you feel. You can only trust information that has been researched properly. How do you know those women really are getting better–that they're healing from their pain as you claim? That's ludicrous. Even those big pain clinics with all their access to data and good scientific studies rarely talk the way you do." And so the rational voice continued and dominated the committee.

Finally, the critical voice interrupted. "Besides–it's enough that you're a regular doctor doing all those regular doctor things. You simply don't have time to be writing and thinking those crazy thoughts. Leave that up to the experts. Look at how you've neglected yourself–you don't exercise enough, don't eat right–shame on you." And then the critical voice went for the jugular. "Besides look at how you neglect your family–you'll pay a price for that."

I listened to the two booming voices on the committee. Finally, they had exhausted their arguments.

And then, the avoidance voice started in. Not terribly loud, but certainly part of the committee. "You're too serious. Look at yourself–no one cares about the stuff you're talking about. Life is to have fun–get with it. Toss out your computer–get some golf clubs. What's wrong with you anyway?"

Oh, to escape, I thought. It's so easy. Why not? I've done it so many times before–do it again. Just disappear. Be silent.

There were others on the committee getting in their stuff. The committee roared in my head. My head ached. My neck felt tense. The pain intensified and I felt my head moving to my neck and rubbing that sore spot.

Ouch. A branch hit my face. I rubbed my eye. I stopped, not knowing where I was. I realized I had been deep in thought. I looked around as the pain in my eye subsided. I felt overwhelmingly tired. I stepped into a clearing. I looked toward the top of the hill and noticed a nice area of grass. I realized I wanted to lie down. I felt too tired to walk further.

I stretched out on the grass. I closed my eyes and felt the sting from the branch subside. I felt the pain in my neck. I felt my tears beginning to flow. I wanted this to be easier.

I waited. I waited more. And then I heard the last committee member. Her voice was quiet. Her voice was barely audible.

"Can you hear me?" she said.

"Yes, I can, but you seem so far away," I said.

"I am far away," the quiet voice said. "You will have to learn to listen to me. It will be hard for you."

"I'm tired," I said. "Part of me wants you to go away. I want this to be easier."

"I know," she said. "You learned your lessons so well. You learned to silence me. You learned to shut me out, because you needed to survive. You learned to speak only the words that they wanted to hear, and that meant you were silenced most of the time. You did not learn to speak your truth. You needed to survive in a world that does not value my quiet voice–the voice of woman, the lost voice. To hear me will take work for you. It will take courage to begin to listen to this lost voice–to learn to hear the voice of the feminine. To learn to believe in who you are and to have the courage to speak your truth will take practice for you," the quiet voice continued.

I stretched on the grass. I rolled my head slowly back and forth. The pain in my head and neck subsided. And slowly, slowly the lost voice became clearer and clearer. I heard the lost voice. I believed and felt whole. Gradually I relaxed. My breathing slowed and became quiet. I rested. The sun shone brightly. The wind blew gently over my face and hair. The birds sang.

Index